No More Crunches
No More Back Pain

The Ab Revolution™

Third edition, Expanded

Dr. Jolie Bookspan

A groundbreaking method to use abdominal
and core muscles functionally –
the way your body needs for healthier daily activity,
exercise, and back pain control

Used by athletes,
military and law enforcement personnel,
and top spine docs and rehab centers

ISBN: 978 0-9721214-2-0

Dedication

To my grandmother the gypsy, who taught me to spot snake oil, and showed me real exercise, body mechanics, and health from my earliest years. She got her college degree at age 81. To her the highest things in life were education and Jack LaLane.

To my mother. I promised her when I was four years old that I would find how to end back pain.

To my students and patients, who all feel better and work their abs more using this method. They showed me how needed it is.

To my wonderful husband and hero, Paul. What beautiful abs you have, my dear.

Table of Contents

Introduction by Andrew Seigel, Second Degree Black Belt

I bought this book after attending a seminar with this extraordinary lady—more on that in a moment. This book is invaluable to anyone who wants to eliminate back-pain immediately. Most of us have been told so many times to "stand up straight, don't slouch" that we do precisely the wrong thing, over-arching and putting strain and stress on our back each and every day. With Dr. Bookspan's straightforward, no-nonsense approach, you can instantly modify a key bad posture and the pain/ache in your lower back IS GONE. What is deceptive is how easy this is to accomplish and so on first read, you might not totally grasp the concept. Take your time with the book, try each modification and exercise as she clearly explains it, and give it a try. Your first goal should be to stop the pain, your second to start strengthening your abs and back by retraining your daily habits - and let me tell you, you'll thank her for it.

As a 40-year-old martial arts instructor with 24 years experience, I was fortunate enough to attend one of her seminars. That's where she really works her magic, face to face. She utilized the concepts in her book to change the way a room full of martial arts instructors and grandmasters live their daily lives. For all of our knowledge and experience, Dr. Bookspan provided a collective epiphany to over 60 veteran martial artists, we were all shaking our heads in amazement and smiling at how good our backs felt. It's practical and it works! To her credit, Dr. Bookspan lives her healthy lifestyle philosophy. This book is not very big, nor is Dr. Bookspan, but both are filled with tremendous power and wisdom. Everyone could benefit from the Ab Revolution.

What is the Ab Revolution™?

_____

1. What is the Ab Revolution?

The Ab Revolution is a revolutionary core training method—no crunches or forward bending. It combines sports medicine with fun exercises. You get a workout at the same time that you retrain your muscles and spine position for healthier movement for all your activities. The Ab Revolution has two components. The first is to learn how to consciously use your core to reposition your spine away from injurious positioning into healthful position for back pain control during everything you do. Lower back and facet pain from hyperlordosis is quickly stopped without doing exercises or strengthening. The second component uses the new healthy positioning during innovative exercises for healthier and more effective exercise than conventional core training.

As a back pain control method, The Ab Revolution is done, not by tightening or exercising, but simply using core muscles to move your spine out of unhealthy position, and to maintain healthy vertebral angle during daily life. As an exercise for fitness, weight loss, and core muscle workout, Ab Revolution exercises can be done in the gym, weight room, at home, and during favorite sports and everyday activities. All the exercises can be put together to music as a hi-energy fitness class.

The Ab Revolution was developed by Dr. Jolie Bookspan, a military scientist, in response to the high incidence of back pain from conventional abdominal exercises, and lack of transfer to daily life.

2. What does The Ab Revolution™ do that conventional abdominal exercises don't?

The Ab Revolution works differently in several ways. It strengthens abdominal and core muscles without forward bending. It specifically teaches healthful spine positioning at the same time as it strengthens. By retraining how to hold neutral spine, it quickly removes a major source of lower back pain without having to do exercises. It provides effective abdominal exercises for those who want exercise, from simple to more challenging than conventional exercises. It dispels myths about abs, and is functional, meaning it trains your muscles to be more effective in the way you move in real life.

Forward bending at the neck, back, and hip for exercise trains rounded posture and is a known factor in neck and back pain, and is counterproductive for most people after a day of sitting.

Strengthening alone will not fix an injury or pain, and will not change injurious body positioning. Plenty of muscular people have pain. Unhealthy spine ergonomics, common during exercise, sports, and daily life, can compress the joints and discs of the back no matter how strong the muscles. The exercises strengthen abdominal and back muscles (simultaneously) while specifically teaching how to use the core muscles to maintain healthful spine position during the exercise, and to transfer that knowledge of positioning to all activities during the rest of your day.

The Ab Revolution dispels old myths, for example, to use abs you must tighten them or "suck them in" or "press your navel to your spine." Tightening does not change injurious spine position or put you into healthy position. You cannot breath in well or move properly when you hold your abdomen tightly. Another myth is that you must keep your knees bent during exercises to "keep your back in proper position." If it were true that you have to bend your knees to protect your back, how are you supposed to stand up and walk away? It is not your knees that position your lower spine, but your abdominal muscles. The Ab Revolution teaches you specifically how to use your abdominal muscles to move your spine and hold it in healthy position.

Another benefit of The Ab Revolution is to put health and fun back into fitness training. "Fitness" is often unhealthy because of fads, emphasis on cosmetic appearance regardless of the toll on the joints, lack of information about how muscles really work, and lack of transferring healthy movement skills to everyday life. The motions and exercises used in The Ab Revolution are functional. That means they train the body and muscles in the way they need to function in real life, standing, and moving, not just when lying on the floor.

3. What Kinds of Back Pain Can The Ab Revolution™ Help?
The techniques directly retrain your core to prevent hyperlordosis (swayback), quickly reversing the facet joint and low back pain that results. Interestingly, someone with reduced lumbar lordosis (flat back) may potentially be helped by Ab Revolution repositioning. The reduced

movement ability of their spine has less tolerance for slouching to end range. Even a small slouch may pressure the less mobile spine. Pain from spondylolisthesis can be quickly diminished by reversing the painfully increased vertebral angle, and improving stability by deliberate positioning. In other populations, hyperlordosis can reduce needed space around spinal nerves and discs, increasing pain from existing conditions such as degenerating/herniated disc, stenosis, and impingement. Some of the bad bending habits creating/worsening these conditions are also addressed in this book. Stop the source and stop the pain.

4. Crunches hurt my neck and sometimes my back. Will Ab Revolution™ exercises hurt my neck?

The forward bending used in conventional abdominal exercise practices and emphasizes forward-rounded posture. Forward bending is hard on your back and neck and does not train how to stand and move when you get up off the floor. The Ab Revolution trains abs without hunching your posture. Many of the exercises are done standing using your muscles to hold straight positioning and neutral spine the way you need for real life. The Ab Revolution trains you how to move in daily life without unhealthy spine positioning that contributes to neck and lower back pain.

5. Does The Ab Revolution™ give you a washboard stomach?

It can. You can work your abs harder with The Ab Revolution™ than with conventional exercises. You work your abs and back at the same time as giving your back healthy definition too. Since The Ab Revolution teaches how to use muscles for real life, you learn to use muscle groups together, a bonus that also works arms and legs and upper body, while getting an ab workout. You can use Ab Revolution exercises together to create a workout to burn calories as part of fat reduction in healthy ways.

6. Who uses The Ab Revolution™?

Anyone who wants to stop lower back pain, improve health, posture, appearance, muscularity, and use of the abdomen and "core" can use The Ab Revolution. The simple pain prevention repositioning can be done by anyone at any fitness level, and is used in the United States and abroad by top spine centers and physicians. Athletes, aerobics instructors and trainers in centers around the world use the exercise techniques for superior training without injury. The toughest components of The Ab Revolution are used by top athletes, law enforcement personnel, military teams, and anyone who wants challenging fun doing abdominal exercise.

7. I have osteoporosis, herniated discs in my neck or back, or Upper Crossed Syndrome. Can I use The Ab Revolution™?

The Ab Revolution does not use forward-rounding and bending exercises. The forward bending of conventional abdominal and core training (crunches, curl-ups, V-sits, "hundreds," and others that bend the spine and hip forward) can put degenerative and herniating forces the discs and are not a good idea for anyone with rounding or fractures from osteoporosis. A habitual rounded forward upper body posture is a main factor in Upper Crossed Syndrome. The Ab Revolution actively retrains muscles away from this posture and problem. Check with your health providers to work sensibly to increase your health and physical abilities using The Ab Revolution.

8. Is it researched as effective?

This method was developed over many years in the lab and in real life with several thousands of students and participants, testing combinations of established and proven sports medicine rehabilitation techniques and physical training methods, then integrating them into real activities. Back pain patients with lordosis and facet pain usually fix their pain from those problems after a single office visit instruction. Ab Revolution functional core retraining was found to relieve lower back pain more effectively than conventional physical therapy (Medicine and Science in Sports and Exercise, Volume 38:5, 2006), and conventional exercises and Pilates (Medicine and Science in Sports and Exercise, Volume 37:5, May, 2005). More work has identified three kinds of hyperlordosis that can be relieved using Ab Revolution techniques (Medicine and Science in Sports and Exercise, Volume 39:5 Supplement May 2007). Ongoing work continues in identifying injury preventing movement technique and healthful core and back strengthening methods.

9. What do medical doctors say about The Ab Revolution™?

"Well, Jolie Bookspan has done it again! An expert at debunking "scientific" bunk, she has developed an extremely effective method that can be used in every day life for the thousands (millions?) who have chronic lumbosacral pain. Freeing the "crunchers" from the boredom of useless exercise programs that are quickly abandoned, the program is simple, sensible, and highly effective. Highly recommended."
—*Ernest Campbell, M.D., FACS, President of the Medical Staff, Chairman of the Department of Surgery, Board of Directors, Brookwood Medical Center*

"I've given *The Ab Revolution* to my physical therapists and trainers to use. You have condensed things to a very workable format."
—*Stanley A. Herring M.D., FACSM, Puget Sound Sports & Spine Physicians, Former President of the North American Spine Society*

"I have learned how to teach patients to treat their back pain. Superb instructor."
—*Fabrice Czarnecki, M.D., Family and Travel Medicine, Hopkins*

"It's about time someone looked at the real science behind the movements, not just mindlessly putting people through the exercises."
—*Thomas M. Bozzuto, D.O., Medical Director Baptist Health System Wound Care Center*

"This is a method that everyone interested in good health and muscle tone should learn- especially trainers!"
—*J. Tom Millington, M.D., Medical Director, St. John's Pleasant Valley Hospital*
"Whenever I have a question on rehab, or want practical advice on fitness training or musculoskeletal complaints, I turn to my friend and colleague, Dr. Jolie Bookspan. I trust her for good sense and her solid background in exercise physiology."
—*David Hsu, M.D., Ph.D., Neurology, Stanford Medical Center*

"If I were to say something sage about exercise, I am afraid that others will die laughing since my aversion to exercise is well known! I always wanted to have you as my personal trainer because you are the only person in the world who might get me to think otherwise about exercise."
—*Caroline Fife, M.D., Associate Professor, Department of Anesthesiology, University of Texas Health Science Center, Houston. Chief Consultant, CHeCS Training Program Krug Life Sciences NASA*

"Dr. Bookspan, the brightest light in popular sports medicine, cuts through the myths and falsehoods about abs."
—*Kelly Hill, M.D., FACSM, Green Beret Lt. Colonel, SWAT Team Commander*

Why is This Method Called a Revolution?
_____

Several aspects make this method a change in thinking about abdominal and core muscles and their role in exercise and back pain prevention.

Abdominal exercise is often thought of as stopping real life to lie on the floor, or use machines, or hunch and bend forward in motions that are not the way you move in real life, but may make your neck hurt and often your back too. The assumption for these exercises is that strengthening the muscles automatically does something to change the lower back or posture. It does not work that way. Strengthening alone does not automatically change posture, prevent the cause of back pain, or teach how you use your muscles in real activities. Many people with strong muscles and tight abs have poor posture, injurious spinal positioning, and persistent back pain.

The Ab Revolution shows how to use abdominal and core muscles to change the positioning of your spine, then applying it to all you do during daily life and exercise. This simple technique is key in how using muscles (not just having them) keeps injurious forces off your back during daily activities while standing up. Conventional ab exercises don't transfer these specific positioning skills to real life. The very thing we regard as exercise advice, "do three sets (or however many sets) of ten crunches," is one of the problems because it separates using your muscles from moving in real life. Ab exercise has become hugely popularized as something you specially "do," then never transfer to the very thing that abs a re supposed to do - hold your spine in neutral, not bent forward or backward. Ab and core exercise is used in many back pain rehabilitation programs but pain often returns because core muscle support to hold you in neutral spine position does not happen automatically from doing bent forward abdominal exercises.

Using abs is also not "tightening" them. You cannot move or breathe properly that way, and tight muscles are a factor in headaches, poor posture, and back pain. Tightening does not move your spine out of unhealthful position into neutral spine. The Ab Revolution does.

The Ab Revolution exercises abdominal and core muscles without crunches or forward bending. It challenges the muscles to hold neutral spine to strengthen them functionally while specifically training you to keep neutral spine during daily life. Conventional forward bending does not teach to use your body the way you need for real life once you get off the floor. In other words, it is not functional. Moreover, crunches, leg lifts, and other forward bending positions can be counterproductive after a day of bending forward over a desk, steering wheel, and everything else.

This method is a change in understanding about abs and their function. This book gives information of what abs really do, what they don't do, and how to consciously use your abs to position your spine and hip for all your activities. It teaches specific skills to make your life better. The exercises strengthen your abdominal muscles, together with your back, arms, shoulders, and legs, and teach you how your muscles need to work together in your real life.

By following the techniques described in this book, you will get exercise without going to a gym. You will strengthen your abdominal muscles without forward bending. You will strengthen your entire body while doing abdominal exercise. You will burn calories. You will stop one of the main injurious postures that creates back pain. You will exercise your brain.

It's a revolution.

Part I
Using the Ab Revolution™ for Back Pain Control

This section is for using abdominal muscles
to maintain neutral spine during ordinary daily life
for back pain control

What Exactly Do Abs Do?

_____

More than other exercises, everyone seems to want to "do abs."
But why?

It's "something" to do with helping your back.
But what exactly do "abs" do for your back?

It's "something" to do with posture.
But exactly what?

It's something vague about "support."
What does "support" really mean?

What do abdominal muscles do?
A prevalent myth is that using abdominal muscles means "sucking them
in" "tightening them" or "pressing navel to spine." You cannot move or
breathe well that way. When you bend your arm, you don't tighten your
muscles to do it. You just move your arm bones using your arm muscles.
Abdominal muscles work the same way. You use them to move the body
parts they attach to.

Abdominal muscles connect your ribs to your hips along your front and
sides. When you use your abs, they pull your ribs and the front of your
hip closer to each other, bending your spine forward to the front or side.

When you stand up and don't use your abs, your ribs and hips move
farther apart. The ribs lift up and/or the hip tips down. Either or both of
these changes in body position exaggerate the normal inward curve of the
lower back. Your lower back sways (over-arches, becoming
hyperlordotic). Over-arching drops the weight of your upper back onto
your lower back, pressing down on your soft tissues and discs, and
eventually irritating the joints called facets where each vertebra attaches to
the next. Much facet pain and injury can result from the simple
unhealthful positioning habit of hyperlordosis (too much inward arch in
the lower spine).

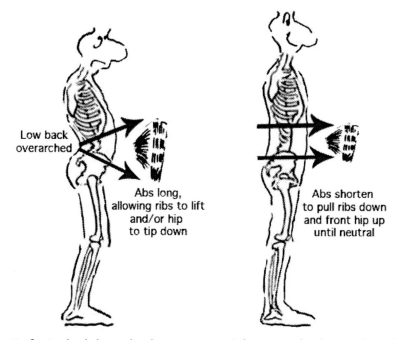

Low back overarched

Abs long, allowing ribs to lift and/or hip to tip down

Abs shorten to pull ribs down and front hip up until neutral

Left: Arched, hyperlordotic posture. The upper body may lean backward, and/or the hip may tilt forward and downward. Both increase the arch, which pressures and pinches the lower back. Right: Returning to neutral spine, using abs to pull ribs down and tuck hip under. A small inward curve remains in the lower back, not a painful exaggerated one.

When does overarching (hyperlordosis) commonly occur? The most common times are during standing. Check and see if you arch your lower back in order to lift your arms or to reach up, and even when you look up. Check and see if you lean back when you carry a load like a laundry basket, chair, or baby. Many people cannot even pull their shoulders back or drink a glass of water without arching their back. Instead of lifting up from the upper body, they arch the lower back. Much "mystery" lower back pain results from the chronic pressure of the arching, but it is just from an easily changed bad posture.

Using your abdominal muscles, just enough to take out excess arching when standing, keeps your upper body weight from pressing backward and downward onto your lower back. You will immediately feel the weight lift off your lower back. Straight positioning does not mean holding yourself rigidly; it means holding yourself up easily and comfortably without slouching backward or to the sides.

Reducing the lower spine arch to neutral to relieve pressure in the lower back is the reason for the footrest in many bars. After long standing at the bar, many people notice that their lower back aches. Putting one foot up on the footrest tucks the hip under a bit, reducing the arch. Back pain reduces immediately. You can do this yourself without the bar using your own abdominal muscles. Moving the spine out of painful position is how abdominal muscles help your back, not through crunches or strengthening the muscles.

Another indirect method to reduce arching and pain is to bend the knees. A common instruction is to stand with bent knees or with one foot in front of the other to reduce pain. Standing arched causes the pain, not foot placement. You can directly reduce the arching by moving your spine with your abdominal muscles, without needing to bend or straighten your knees. Instead of strange rules about standing in bent ways, use your abdominal muscles to reduce the painfully arched position and return to comfortable neutral spine.

Pressure and arching is made worse when the front of the hip is tight. Anterior hip tightness makes it difficult or uncomfortable to stand without overarching when the legs are straight. This means the person is too tight to merely stand up. However, keeping knees bent perpetuates the tightness, and is not a functional way to walk around or get anything done. The issue of "When You Can't Lie Flat Without A Pillow" plus stretching to relieve hip tightness so that you can stand up straight is covered at the end of Part I, pages 44 to 46.

Most people only exercise their abs by hunching forward and sideways for a bunch of "repetitions." Then they stand and walk away not using their abs, allowing their back to arch in the same way that caused pain in the first place. The Ab Revolution shows you how to use your abs while you are standing to reduce the excessive arch. You will stop pain and get a free, built-in abdominal muscle workout at the same time.

What is Lordosis and What is Neutral Spine?

Many people have never heard of lordosis, but have mysterious back pain. They may have been diagnosed with various back issues, but treatments fail, or only partially work, because lordosis was not considered. Others with back pain are sometimes told they have a "condition" called lordosis, also called hyperlordosis or "swayback." It may be described as something anatomic or unavoidable, or the way they were born. Lordosis is not a structural condition. It is how you stand.

Technically, the word "lordosis" originally meant the normal inward curve of the lower back. Lordosis has commonly come to mean excess inward curve, synonymous with hyperlordosis. Excessive lordosis (same as overarching) drops the weight of your upper body down on your lower back. It can create much back pain, but is just a bad posture habit.

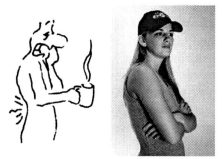

Lordotic (overly arched) spine position
lets upper body weight press downward on the lower back.

Lordosis is often, unfortunately, thought of as normal, or relaxed, or cute. It is not healthy and not normal, even though common. An overly arched, lordotic posture is seen in an astonishing number of fitness videos, magazines, books, and classes. The model may say "keep neutral spine," along with the usual (but incorrect) "tighten your abs." However, you may see that they arch their back and stick out their behind in many exercises such lifting weights, holding a "plank," using the exercise ball, during leg lifts, and other exercises. Allowing the lower spine to slouch and arch under body weight is a weak, unfit posture, is injurious to the lower back, and is a marker of not using abdominal muscles.

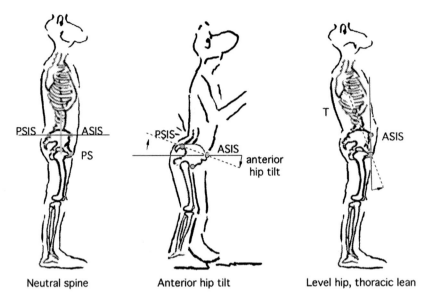

Neutral spine   Anterior hip tilt   Level hip, thoracic lean

In general, (this interesting topic can be involved) think of a line through the crest of your hipbone from back to front. The line from the top bump in back (medical abbreviation is PSIS) to the top bump in front (ASIS) should be approximately horizontal (left). This is neutral spine. A small inward curve remains. If you let your spine slouch so that the front of the hip (ASIS) drops downward (the back tilts outward in back), the small normal inward curve of the lower back increases (middle). The spine is no longer neutral. It is over-arched. Another way to see the anterior hip tilt is in the line from the ASIS to where the pelvic bones meet in front, called the symphysis pubis (PS). When you hold your spine neutral, the line from ASIS to PS is vertical, as is the line from the top of the upper leg bone to the middle of the hip crest (left). When the ASIS tilts forward of the PS and the behind sticks out in back (middle), this is an anterior tilt to the hip. The spine is no longer neutral. It is arched and hyperlordotic. In a second kind of hyperlordosis, the hip may be level, but if you push the hip forward and/or lean the upper body backward, the lower spine increases the arch and becomes pinched under upper body weight.

Hyperlordosis is usually completely controllable by using abs to curl your lower spine forward just enough to return to neutral spine and reduce the overly large arch that makes the lower back painful (left drawing).

Try This To Feel How Abdominal Muscles Control Posture and Reduce the Back Pain of Lordosis

A common assumption is that doing abdominal exercise to strengthen the abs will change your posture or stop back pain. However, strengthening does not do either automatically.

You have to voluntarily use your abdominal muscles to change your positioning to stop back pain. It is just like using arm muscles to move your arm to touch your head. Your arm does not automatically lift up just from having strong arm muscles. You have to deliberately use the muscles. In the same way, if you don't consciously use your abdominal muscles to hold your spine in neutral position, you may sag. That is one big reason people slouch. They aren't using their core muscles to prevent it.

To feel for yourself how abdominal muscles change your posture, try this:

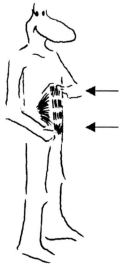

Stand up and put one hand on the front of your ribs where your front abdominal muscles attach (top arrow).

Put your other hand on the front of your hipbone where your front abdominal muscles (rectus muscles) begin (bottom arrow).

The distance between your hands roughly represents abdominal muscles.

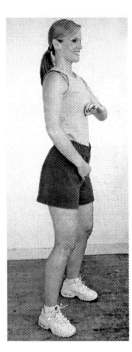

To feel for yourself how not using abdominal muscles increases back pain, try this:

While still holding your ribs and hipbone, let your ribs lift, backside tilt back, and abdomen curve out to arch your lower back. The distance between your hands increases, showing how slack abdominal muscles allow your back to arch.

Let your upper body weight sink backward and downward. Do you feel the pressure in your lower back? This is how lack of use of abdominal muscles allows upper body weight to press down on the lower back, making it hurt.

When standing arched, without using abdominal muscles, you will even be shorter because of the excessive low back curve.

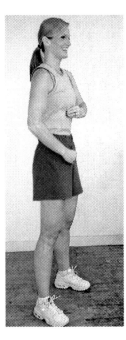

Now try this to feel how abdominal muscles work to reduce lower back pain:

While still standing with your lower back arched, bring your hands toward each other so that the distance between ribs and hips decreases. Your torso pulls forward and upright to a straightened, taller position. A slight inward curve in the lower back remains, but the overly large arch is reduced, producing neutral spine.

Don't bend forward; just stand upright. The pressure in your lower back should be gone. This demonstrates how abdominal muscles control posture and low back pain. When used properly, abdominal muscles keep you from arching backward, and stop the pressure and wear and tear of dropping your upper body weight on your lower back. This only occurs when you deliberately use them to position your spine.

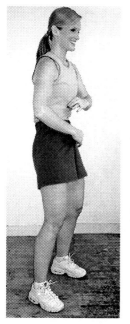

Now, visualize what crunches do:

Still holding the top and bottom of your abdominal muscles, draw your two hands closely toward each other.

Your torso will curl and your back will round forward so that you stoop forward.

Hold that position. That is what crunches do. Are you happy? Does your back feel good or "supported?"

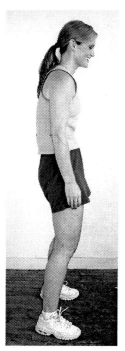

Crunches hunch you forward. How much do you need this posture in real life? Hunching forward for exercise is not highly functional.

Instead of doing crunches and forward bending abdominal exercises, use your abdominal muscles all the time to pull your spine forward just enough to produce neutral spine and stop the overly-arched position that causes pain.

By holding straight position instead of rounding, you will train healthy posture at the same time that you get a free built-in abdominal muscle workout all day.

Try This to Visualize How Abs Work to Reduce Low Back Pain

People usually have a vague idea that abs have something to do with helping the back, but they don't know specifically what abs do, or that abs don't do it automatically. You may have the strongest abs and never use them to stop the arching that causes pain. Here is another way to see what abdominal muscles do to help your back:

Hold your right hand up with your thumb toward you. Your palm (facing left) represents the front of your body. The back of your hand (facing right) is your back. Curl your fingers forward to represent your abs at work. Lift your fingers back up again to simulate using your back muscles to straighten up. Relate this to curling and straightening your body.

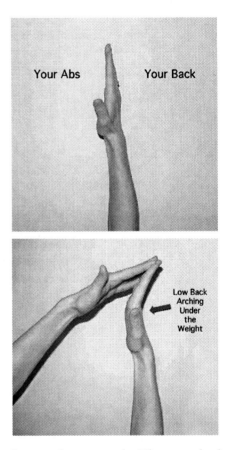

With your left hand, press against the fingers of your right hand, bending your fingers back as far as they will go. Keep your palm upright; only your fingers arch back. See and feel the pinched and folded-back crease at the knuckle joints of your right hand.

Pushing your fingers backward and downward shows how your upper body weight pushes backward and downward on the joints of your low back when you allow your low back to arch too much. The stretched palm of your hand represents your abdomen, with your ab muscles slack and not pulling enough to hold you straight.

Bounce against your fingers so that they rock backward repeatedly. The backward pressing shows the forces on your low back when you walk without using abdominal muscles to prevent overarching. That kind of pressure is what you are doing to your low back every day when you don't consciously use your abs to prevent overarching. If you bounce against your fingers quickly and firmly, you can imagine the effect of running with your lower back allowed to overarch. Ouch.

To represent how your abs can prevent overarching, try this: With your left hand still pressing the right-hand fingers backward, use the muscles in the palm of your right hand to straighten your right hand against the push of your left. Your fingers come back up into a straight line. That is how you need to use abs to control your posture when standing. It's not tightening the muscles or strengthening, just using them to move your spine to prevent pain.

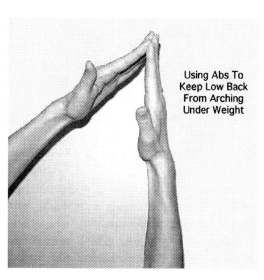

Using Abs To Keep Low Back From Arching Under Weight

Now you know how to prevent the overly large lower back arch (hyperlordosis) that creates back pain: you use abdominal muscles to pull your spine forward enough to return to neutral spine. And healthful upright posture Don't pull forward so much that you hunch or round your upper body forward, or push your hip forward of your body.

Can You Stand Upright Without Overarching?

A surprising number of people are so round-shouldered that they cannot stand straight without arching their back. To bring their head up and shoulders back, they arch their back instead of straightening their upper body from the upper body and shoulders. Try this:

- Stand against a wall with your heels, hips, and shoulders touching the wall.

- Bring the back of your head against the wall. That is where your head should be for healthful posture, even when you are relaxed.

- Did you let your ribs come up and your back arch? Fix that by using your abdominal muscles to tuck the hip under, as if starting a "crunch" just enough to reduce the overarch back to neutral.

If your upper back and shoulders are so stiff that you cannot stand up straight without arching your back, try stretching the front muscles of your chest (pectoral muscles). One quick, easy, chest (pectoral) stretch is to face a wall with one elbow bent to the side at about 90 degrees. The inside of your elbow touches the wall. Turn your feet and body away from the elbow using the wall to brace and pull the elbow backward. Keep shoulder relaxed down. Make sure you feel the stretch in your front chest muscles, not your shoulder joint.

Tight chest muscles pull the upper body into round-shouldered position. Many traditional stretches make you more round-shouldered by rounding forward. Avoid them, along with pulling one arm over your chest in front, which further encourages round-shouldered position. Instead, use stretches that pull your upper body backward, not rounded forward. A good stretch book resource is listed at the end of this book.

To practice straight, relaxed head and upper back posture, stand against a wall or lie flat without a pillow under your knees or head. A small inward curve remains in your lower back, but not a large one. During the day, practice keeping your shoulders back without arching your back to do it.

What About the Ab Study?

A fitness industry survey compared 13 of the most common abdominal exercises and ranked them from most to least effective in producing ab muscle activity. It is a common assumption that weak abs are somehow connected to back pain, so it is often concluded that therefore strengthening the muscles is what is needed. This approach hasn't been working. There are several reasons why:

- An exercise may exercise a muscle, yet at the same time promote injurious posture and not be good for the rest of you. Just as smoking "works" to lose weight, crunches and forward-rounding abdominal exercises "work" the abs but are not a healthful way to do it.

- Even if an exercise activates abdominal muscles, it still may not be useful for how you move in daily life. You don't hunch forward for daily activities. You do need your abs to help you to stand and walk upright without arching and sagging backward. Crunches and other exercises tested in the study don't train that. Posture and muscle use are not automatic. Just strengthening a muscle does not train it for how you need it to work.

- Strengthening abdominal muscles will not automatically change spine positioning for healthy use in sports and recreation, or for back pain control. Plenty of muscular people have poor posture and much back pain.

The Ab Revolution teaches a different approach to abdominal muscle use, gives exercises that effectively develop your abs, and shows you how to transfer use of abdominal and other core muscles to daily life. Even if you don't care about posture or back pain and want only the cosmetic results of strong abs, use the Ab Revolution exercises in Part II for effective workouts.

What's Wrong with Crunches?

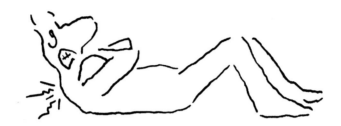

Crunches don't work your core muscles the way you need for real life. Crunches don't train your core to hold your spine in position the rest of the day. Crunches promote poor posture, even when done properly.

Look at crunches sideways and see what it would look like to stand up like this — like an old, bent-over person. How did many bent-over people became like that? They practiced. They spent their life rounding their spine until it became deformed and stuck rounded. Bent forward rounding is the same problematic posture that crunches train.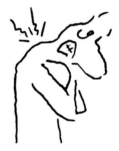

The most important use of abdominal muscles is when you are standing , carrying things, and reaching or lifting overhead. Most people cannot imagine how to use their abs while standing up or during normal everyday life. In life, your abs need to work isometrically — at one length — to hold your torso upright, instead of allowing you to arch back. Crunches don't train you for that. Crunches make people, who likely spend much of their day already hunched over a work area, practice that hunched posture, which may be mechanically promoting the back and neck pain they think they are working their abs to prevent. No wonder that doing 10 minutes of "abs" a day cannot counteract the other 23 hours and 50 minutes a day of non-use and wrong use.

Doing conventional abdominal exercise does not change arched bad posture. This is why most conventional ab exercises don't stop back pain. People do crunches all the time but don't know they are supposed to use their ab muscles in real life when standing to prevent over-arching.

Doing Ab Exercise Doesn't Automatically Change Posture, Vertebral Angle, or Lower Back Pain

If you strengthen your arm muscles, the strong muscles don't automatically hold your arm up in the air, or "support" your arm. In the same way, strengthening your abdominal muscles does not make them automatically do anything to support your back. You have to deliberately use your abdominal (and other posture muscles, including back muscles) to adjust your spine position yourself. This is why doing crunches, yoga, or rehab exercises—as exercises without the knowledge to deliberately position during real activities —does not often work as expected.

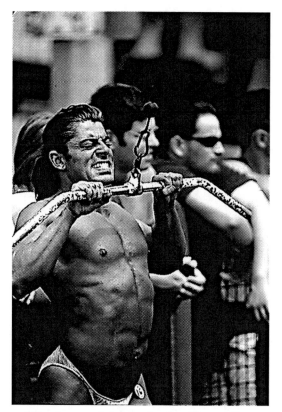

His abs are tight yet he is still standing
in poor posture with an overly arched lower back.
Having tight abs does not automatically fix posture or help your back.

Overly arched positioning causes back pain and reduces the effectiveness of many exercises. See for yourself. When you try the "pull-down" exercise on page 23, keep your hip tucked and stand upright without arching backward to pull the weight down. You will feel a far more effective exercise, and you will feel your abdominal muscles working hard to control spine positioning and prevent the spine from arching.

Doing abdominal exercises or core exercises is not like getting a shot of penicillin or going to confession. It does not "fix" things. Using abdominal muscles is like toilet training. You need to learn what to do, make your mistakes until you remember, then hold it even when you don't feel like it.

Abdominal muscle use is conscious, deliberate use to move your torso away from arching and into healthy position, just like using any other voluntary muscles to move any other part of your body. If you don't, no matter how muscular you are, or how many crunches you have done, you can still wind up with poor spinal position, bad posture, and back pain.

Spondylolisthesis. A spinal condition called spondylolisthesis makes one lower vertebra slip forward on the next, adding to back arching and lordosis. If you have spondylolisthesis, it becomes even more important to use The Ab Revolution to hold your spine in position during all your daily activities.

Aren't You Supposed to Stick Your Behind Out?

In some cases, people deliberately push their behind out in back, thinking that the unhealthful posture looks cute or sexy, similar to believing that smoking a cigarette looks good, rather than unhealthy. In other cases, programs teach to stick far out in back, in effort to avoid opposite problem of tucking too much and rounding forward, which contributes to back pain and disc injury. However, overcompensating by over-arching backward is also unhealthful. Initially, overarching backward seems to "work" since you can lift more because you shift some of the work off your muscles and onto your lower spine. The muscles do less, so the lift seems easier. Competition lifters use it to lift more, regardless of the pain and injuries it causes later on. Instead, use the hip tuck, just enough to return to neutral spine and avoid overarching, to shift effort to core muscles and off the lower back. You don't need to overarch backward to prevent the problems of too much forward rounding.

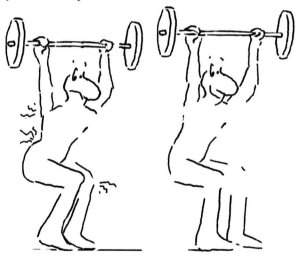

Don't overarch (left). Use the hip tuck to straighten enough to
return to neutral spine to prevent overpressuring the lower back (right).

Another problem during squatting exercises is rocking forward, shifting body weight to the knee joint. This is common when Achilles tendons are tight. Keep heels down and knees over heels (right drawing), which shifts weight from knee joints to leg muscles.

Rounding the spine forward under the weight of your body or external weights pressures the lower vertebral discs. That is why it is not healthful to bend forward to lift things, or sit or stand with your back rounded. The vertebrae press together in front and open in back. Over years of pressing, the discs begin to move outward to the back, like squeezing a tube of toothpaste. Finally one day after years of abuse, a low back disc can finally squeeze out enough to hurt. It feels sudden, but like a heart attack from narrowed blood vessels, it was building for years. Low back muscles and discs are pressured through bending with both a rounded and straight back. The dynamics are a little different, but in short, it is healthier and more exercise to bend right with a good upright squat or lunge. Books explaining more are listed at the back of this book.

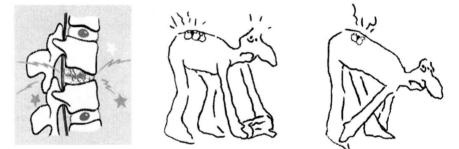

Left: Spine segment showing how bending forward presses discs out toward the back. Right: Years of forward bending can pressure discs outward enough to degenerate and herniate them.

Lifting properly with an upright torso, instead of bending over, protects your back and discs by shifting the load off your discs and onto the leg and back muscles. Similarly, using Ab Revolution repositioning to reduce excessive low back arch when standing and lifting overhead, protects your back and spinal joints by shifting the load off the low back and onto the abdominal and core muscles.

Ab Revolution exercises strengthen without spinal rounding that pressures discs, and it teaches functional use of abs in the same healthy straight positioning needed to stop back pain during daily life and exercise.

Problems From Overarching (Hyperlordosis)

An overly arched (lordotic) posture is unhealthy for several reasons:
- Without using abdominal muscles to keep the spine from overarching, the weight of your upper body and everything you lift and carry presses downward on your lower back. The compression eventually hurts the joints of the spine called facets, surrounding soft tissue, and puts degenerating forces on the discs.

- Arching changes the tilt of your hip, interfering with normal walking and running mechanics. Your hips endure extra wear. Keeping the muscles in front of your hip in a shortened position tightens them, causing a cycle of tightness, poor posture, poor use, and pain.

- Arching is sloppy technique and wasted effort because it does not effectively employ abdominal muscles. Why spend time exercising when you don't get benefit? You are missing a free workout of your core muscles.

- Arching is a sign that you are not generating effective force in your limbs during arm or leg activity, because core muscles are not driving the limbs. See the sections on punching and kicking.

Overarched posture of the lower back and a forward-tilted hip (photo at right) is accepted as normal so often that it is mistaken for, even used to advertise, for fitness and trimness. However, overarching is a sign of a tight hip, of not using abdominal muscles, and is a frequent and often missed contributor to lower back pain.

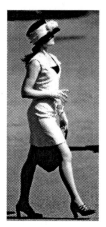

Advertising uses overarched bad posture because sex sells. So does heroin. There is no excuse to display a lack of health, yet call it fitness. Notice when you see "fitness" models standing or exercising with unhealthy overarched posture. You may notice often, because this unfit posture is a pervasive problem.

How to Use Abs When Standing to Stop Low Back Pain– (How to Learn Neutral Spine)

Many people cannot imagine using their abs when standing normally. Using core muscles when standing to move the spine to neutral is how to stop the source of hyperlordotic lower back pain, and better use your core during activities. Following are a few ways to learn neutral spine. Try them all until one (hopefully all) make sense, and you understand how to move your spine out of arched position into neutral. None of the following are exercises to do ten times, or every day, they are just concepts to understand how to move your spine into neutral. Then you use the knowledge of how to move to neutral during all you do.

Method 1 - Visual With Hands. Use the technique on page 16. Start out standing arched with your hands on each end of your abs. Contract your abs so that your ribs and hip, with hands, draw closer, reducing hyperlordotic (overarched) position back to neutral spine.

Method 2 - Thumbs. Stand with hands on hips, thumbs to the back and fingers over the front of the hipbone. Roll your hip so that your thumbs roll downward in back. Don't overtilt or push the hip forward.

Method 3 - Standing Crunch. Do an abdominal crunch while standing. Feel the bottom of your hip swing under. Feel your ribs pull downward and forward. Do this just enough to stand upright and straight, not curled forward. A small inward curve remains in the lower back.

Method 4 - Wall Push. Stand with your back against a wall. Press your lower back toward the wall. Don't completely flatten against the wall, just feel the hip tilt needed to bring the lower back closer to the wall. It will be like the standing crunch in Method 2. The back of the hip rotates under until it no longer sticks out in back, and is straight under you.

Method 5 - Hands and Knees. Kneel on all fours. Lift and round your back upward, feeling your behind lower and tuck under.

Method 6 - Floor Pelvic Tilt. Lie on your back on the floor. Begin to press your lower back toward the floor. This is the "pelvic tilt. " The pelvic tilt is often misunderstood and given as a back pain reduction exercise. Doing a number of tilts is not what helps the back. The use of the tilt is to know what to do when you stand up, to prevent overarching. The pelvic tilt is not a back exercise to do 10 times, it is something to do once - all the time when standing. Don't overtilt.

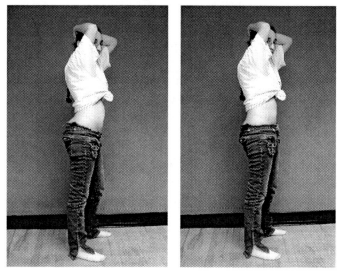

Left: The lower back is overly arched and hyperlordotic. The beltline tips down in front. Right: Restoring neutral spine by tucking the bottom of the hip under to straight position. Belt line becomes level.

Now Test It In Use. Reach high up overhead. Did your ribs lift and your back arch? Did you let your hips move forward or tip down in front? Many people arch their back every time they reach. That drops weight on their low back each time. Eventually the low back starts to hurt. While still reaching overhead, tuck your hip and pull your upper body forward until straight. If you use the hip tuck correctly, you will immediately feel pressure disappear from your lower back. Feel a new strong feeling in your torso. Keep this new healthier posture all the time.

Use the Ab Revolution whenever you stand and reach overhead—from pulling off shirts, to reaching cabinets, to washing hair, to lifting weights and babies overhead. You will save your back, improve your posture, be able to lift more, and get a free all-day workout just from standing and doing your life with your muscles in use.

Using "Upper and Lower Abs" When Standing to Stop Low Back Pain

There is much discussion about what determines "upper" and "lower" abs, what exercises "work" them, or even if upper and lower abs exist. The words upper and lower refer to abdominal muscle fibers that are higher or lower in the body, not separate muscles. In that context, there are no separate "upper" or "lower" muscles. However, the different areas of the whole muscle do pull differently and the upper and lower body can slouch differently to produce several ways to overarch. Try the following to understand how muscles produce movement and how that changes spine positioning.

Upper abs (or upper body thoracic lean)
One way the spine becomes overly-lordotic is to allow the upper body to sag and lean backward. Some people also let the hip push forward. The solution is to pull the upper body forward until you are straight. Don't tuck the hip in this case, since it is already too far forward.

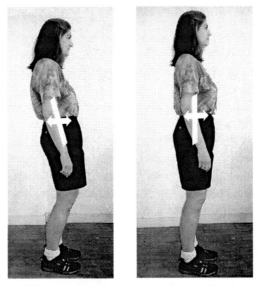

Left: Hip pushed forward and upper body sagging backward, which increases lower back arch. Right: Corrected by pulling the upper body forward to straight position.

Watch other people and see when they lean back or tilt their hip forward in front when walking, doing biceps curls, lifting weights, reaching overhead, taking photos, and many other activities. They are not using "upper" abs, they are missing a free ab workout, and they are adding to strain and wear on their back.

Lower abs
Not using the lower position of the abdominal muscles fibers (and oblique abdominal muscles) lets the front of the hip tilt downward. The behind tips out in back. If the front of your hip is tight, you may arch your lower back like this to lift up the upper body to stand straight. This arching is hard on the back and hip.

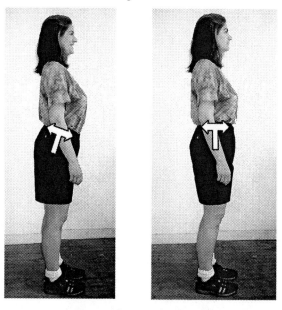

Left: Poor position not using "lower abs." Beltline tilts down in front. Hip is tilted forward from the top of the leg bone to the middle of the hip. Behind tips out in back. Low back is arched. Right: Corrected to neutral by tucking the hip under and leveling the beltline.

To fix lower body overarching, tuck your hip under so that the front of your hip straightens where it meets your leg (right). You will feel a slight upward stretch in the front of the hip. Don't lean back or jut the hip forward. Just tuck enough to pull yourself into upright posture. You will feel your lower abs pulling your front, lower hipbone upward and inward.

Notice when people tilt their hip and stick their hip and behind out when walking, taking aerobics and step class, stretching, lifting weights, and during other activities. They are not using their abdominal muscles they are missing a free ab workout, and they are adding to strain and wear on their back. Correct this posture and you will use your "lower abs" in an all-day "reverse crunch."

Both upper and lower body overarching
Not using abs all along their length lets the upper body sway backward and the hip tilt downward in front. The abdomen curves out and the behind juts out in back.

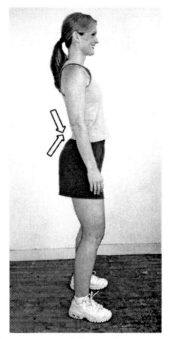

Overarched spine, without control from the upper or lower torso muscle. The front of the hip tilts forward, the behind tips out in back, and the upper body leans backward.

To use your abdominal muscles to fix upper and lower body position, bring your behind forward just enough to bring it to a straight position by tucking your hip under. The front crease of your hip straightens where it meets your leg. Pull the upper body forward until you are straight.

Don't round forward. Just use your muscles to stand straight in relaxed healthy position

Fixing low back positioning (posture) using upper abs and lower abs
This section explained how there is a "not using upper abs" bad posture, a "not using lower abs" bad posture, and combinations of the two. All are unhealthy for your back. They are sloppy postures because they do not use abdominal muscles for healthy standing. It's a shame that unhealthy standing position has become mistaken for an attractive or relaxed stance.

When you notice your back hurts when you are standing around, notice if you are arching. You may be standing with your upper body leaning back with your hips forward, or your low back arched and your behind stuck out in back. Reposition yourself. Correct and straighten your positioning and you will burn more calories, stand taller, and get free, all-day exercise for "upper and lower" abs.

Using Abs Doesn't Mean "Sucking Them In" or Making Them "Tight"

Using your abs does not mean "sucking them in,"
or "tightening them,"
or "pressing your navel to your spine."

Tightening and pressing are practically universal phrases to describe using abdominal muscles, yet they are incorrect and outdated. They are not the way to use your abs the way you need for real life movement.

Tightening is not how to use abs, or any muscles, for good posture. You can have poor posture, back pain, and an overly-arched back, even with "tight" abs.

To see why tightening is not how to use abs, try this:
Bend your elbow to bring your hand up to your face. You didn't tighten anything.

Now move your arm around. It didn't tighten. You voluntarily move your arm into the position you want by using the muscles, not tightening them. Now move your torso side to side, then forward and back. You didn't tighten, you just used abdominal and core muscles. Moving your torso into good posture by using your core muscles is the same. It is just voluntary movement to change the amount of bend and arch in your spine.

Now try tightening your abdominal muscles, as commonly taught. Press your navel to your spine. Tighten the entire area. Now while holding tight, breathe in. You can't. Note that such tightening would not be possible or useful for daily activity. Moreover, walking around with "tight" muscles is a common factor in headache and stress/strain-related muscle pain.

Next stand with arched posture. Tighten your abs and surrounding musculature. Note that posture does not change.

Now stop tightening the area so that movement is unrestricted. Tuck your spine and hip to remove the lordotic arch, straightening your posture. Now you see that "using your abs" means moving them, just like any other muscle, to move your body.

Instead of lying on the floor and hunching forward to exercise your abs, train your abs to work the way you really need them—standing up.

By using your abs to hold healthy spine positioning during all your activities, you will get free exercise and ab training that benefits your life and helps your back. Simply strengthening abs will not help your back. Using them to keep healthy torso posture is how it works.

Yes, this is new and different. That's why it's a revolution in ab and core fitness. It will change your entire way of thinking about abs, and teach you exciting new skills to be fitter, healthier, and pain free.

How to Prevent Low Back Pain When Reaching and Lifting Overhead

People often arch their back when the reach up. They lean back instead of extending the shoulder. To see how this arching often occurs, try this:

- Stand up and reach high overhead with both hands. Did your ribs come up and your back arch?

- Now bring your upper body forward until you are straight. Use your abs as if you were beginning a crunch but not curling forward or bending your neck. This is how to use abs to reach. Reducing the arch keeps strain off the low back and gives better use of the shoulder.

- You may notice that your arm does not reach as high as before. While holding tucked, straight spine and hip position, stretch up from the shoulder. You will get a batter shoulder stretch.

Picture this: someone with shoulder pain goes to the doctor who asks them to reach overhead. They arch their back and reach their hand straight to the ceiling. They are checked as having normal shoulder range of motion. What really happened was that they arched their back when lifting their arm. Their shoulder really did not stretch as much as needed.

Now picture people arching when reaching all day, every day, for shelves, packages, groceries, lifting the baby, combing hair, pulling off shirts, and at the gym to lift weights.

Using abdominal muscles to maintain healthy spine position gives you the opportunity to get more range of motion in your shoulders, more exercise for your abs, and the direct way to stop the overarching pressure that causes low back pain.

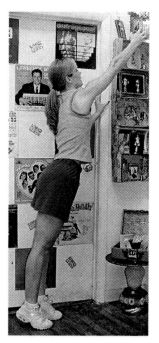 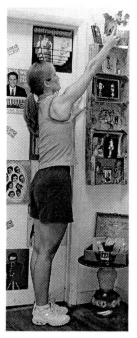

Left: Back arched, abs not in use. Right: Using abdominal muscles
to tuck the hip under and straighten lower back posture.

Now try this technique with hand weights and packages

- Lift weights high overhead. See if you let your back arch to raise your arms.

- Instead of letting your low back arch, keep your abdominal muscles in use to prevent arching, as if beginning a crunch, but not curling forward or bending your neck.

- Keep your hip tucked under you, not sticking out in back or pushed forward. Stand straight, not tightly, just in a healthy and relaxed manner.

- Feel the effort shift to your abdominal muscles. The pressure in the lower back should be gone.

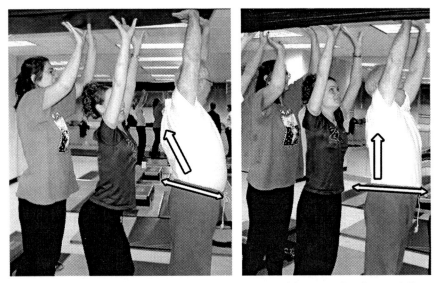

Left photo: Student on far left is arching and leaning back. Middle student is arching and tilting forward. Man on right tips the hip down in front and the upper body backward. Right photo: Corrected positioning. Note how the hips become level.

Transfer the exercise of keeping healthy torso posture to real life. Use it when reaching and lifting weight overhead for common activities like lifting bags, trays, cargo onto on car roof racks, heavy packages onto counters, putting away groceries, lifting babies and children overhead, and whenever you lift and reach.

How to Use The Ab Revolution™ to Prevent Low Back Pain When Carrying Loads in Front

When carrying anterior loads, it is common to arch back to offset the load. Arching shifts the weight to your lower back. Remember not to lean the upper body backward, push the hip forward, or tilt the hip. Maintain upright position and neutral spine against the pull of the load, with whatever you carry in front of you. You will feel your abs working to do this.

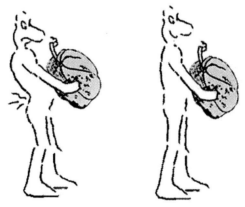

Left: Arched (lordotic) lower spine posture. The upper back is leaning backward and the hip is tilting forward. Don't arch back to offset the weight of an anterior load. Instead, use neutral spine (right).

When carrying or lifting any load in front, from groceries, to a chair, to a pregnancy, or a baby on your hip, don't lean back to offset the load. To stop the arching and the lower back pain that results, tuck your hip under you, as if doing a small abdominal crunch standing up, until you are straight without rounding forward. Don't over-tuck, tighten, round your shoulders, or lean forward or backward. Just stand straight. When you tuck properly by moving your spine (not by tightening anything) the too-large arch will lessen to normal, and pressure in your lower back from the arching should immediately disappear.

It may be tempting to rest a carried weight on your hip and lean back, letting your low back take the brunt. Instead, get free arm and ab exercise.

How to Use The Ab Revolution™ to Prevent Low Back Pain During Pregnancy

Lack of use of abdominal muscles to prevent hyperlordosis is common during pregnancy. Leaning the upper body back and letting the hip tilt forward brings with it much low back pain. Hyperlordosis is not caused by a pregnant belly, or even a beer belly. The over-arching (hyperlordosis) is not unchangeable anatomy. It is leaning back to offset the load in front.

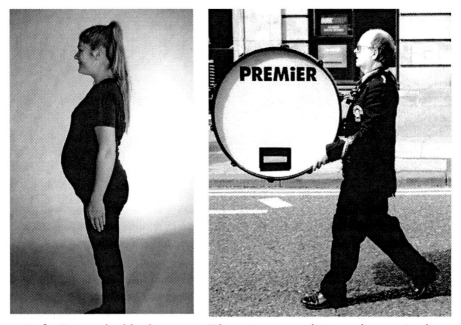

Left: Overarched bad posture. There is too much inward curve in the lower back. Carrying a pregnancy is like carrying any other anterior load; don't arch back to offset the weight. Right: Posture is upright with neutral spine, not arched against the anterior load.

Increased lordosis is not an unavoidable consequence of pregnancy. It is a lack of using abs. Of all times to use your abs to prevent the common change in back posture and the back pain that results, this is it.

How to Use The Ab Revolution™ to Prevent Low Back Pain When Carrying Loads on Your Back and to the Sides

It is not the case that you should not carry shoulder bags or a backpack because they make you arch your back. Backpacksdo not make you arch your back. You arch when you allow the weight to pull you into an arch. It is common to lean back or to the side under the weight of a bag. Instead, straighten up. Don't allow your lower back to be pulled backward into an arch under the load. Pull your upper body forward if you are allowing the backpack to pull your upper body back. If you are sticking your behind out in back to rest the weight of the pack, tuck the hip back under you. You will feel your abdominal muscles working to hold you straight against the load. Try this:

- Stand up wearing any heavy book bag or backpack. Stand sideways to see your profile in a mirror. Let the bag pull your upper body backward. You may feel pressure or a familiar ache in your lower back. (Don't do this if you have back pain.)

- Fix your spine positioning by pulling your upper body forward and bringing your hips under as if starting a crunch. Bring the upper body forward until you are straight, not rounding or hunching forward. Feel your torso straighten against the pull of the bag. You should feel the back pain disappear.

Remember to use abdominal and back muscles to hold torso posture upright without leaning forward or arching back against the pull of the load with everything you carry. Use. Your bags, babies, and other things carried become a free core muscle workout. People go to a gym to strap a weight machine onto their back to pull it forward to work their muscles. Your bags become free, built-in abdominal exercise.

Check your posture with a mirror when you can. Practice walking around carrying things, maintaining upright posture, not bent in any direction against the load.

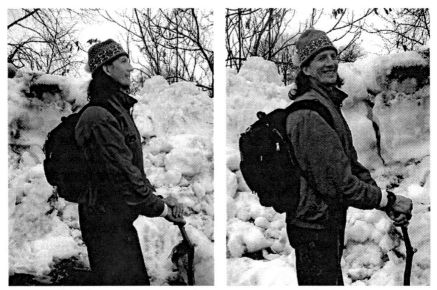

Left: Back is arched against the posterior load, shifting the weight of
the backpack to the lower back. Right: Abs are in use to keep
the lower back from arching, relieving strain.

Shoulder bags and babies carried on the hip

If you habitually let your spine curve to the side under the weight of
things you carry instead of simply holding good posture by using your
muscles, you can eventually tighten your back and even deform your
bones into a curve. Even if you don't have scoliosis, an abnormal
sideways curve, you can get a similar curve from bad posture. This is
preventable.

Fix your posture by engaging your oblique abs (side ab muscles) to
straighten your torso against the sideways pull of whatever you carry. Try
this wearing a knapsack, holding a baby, or carrying a heavy handbag on
one shoulder or hip: Experiment with the difference between maintaining
upright posture and letting your body sag to the side or lifting your
shoulder against the weight.

Using Abs to Prevent Back Pain When Swimming and Scuba Diving

Although swimming is a common prescription for back pain patients, it is also common to increase low back pain through unhealthful positioning while swimming and scuba diving. A commonly held belief is that swimming the front crawl "makes you arch your back." However, swimming does not make you arch, it is you allowing it. If you do not prevent overarching, whether from craning to look up, to kick, or when legs float upward, the fulcrum of the kick becomes the lower back joints instead of the muscles of the abdomen, back, and hip.

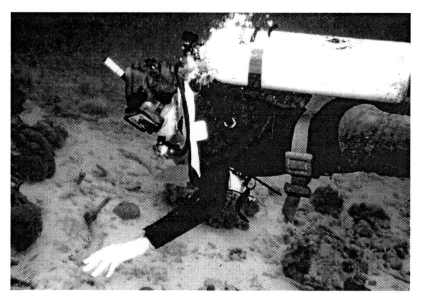

Avoid overarching the lower back and/or hiking the back of the hip upward, as in the photo above, when swimming and scuba diving.

The same principles of using abdominal muscles when standing and doing other movement apply to swimming. Use core muscles to straighten spine positioning. Reducing overarching gives better streamline, a more powerful kick, and stops the pressure and pain of "creasing" the low back by arching.

When You Can't Lie Flat Without A Pillow

Many people keep their hip bent all day, then sleep with a pillow under their knees at night. They rarely straighten their hip. They stand and walk bent at the hip. Vicious cycles form from doing exercises and activities of daily living (ADLs) with the hip bent (flexed), which tightens it, and tight hips forcing a flexed posture. Inability to extend the hip to a straight position creates a flexed posture and an arched lower back.

Your hip flexors are the muscles that bend your leg forward at the hip. When they are tight, it may become uncomfortable to lie flat on the floor. As the tight hip pulls back into arch, it pinches the low back. Using a pillow under the knees all the time only keeps the hip tight and bent. The remedy is to stretch the hip, not put a pillow under knees, which keeps hip flexed and perpetuates problem, not solves it.

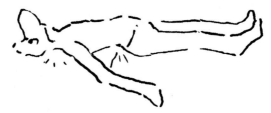

The same problem of pain from tightness causing arching can occur when lying face down. Pain coming from a tight hip when lying face down has given rise to the mistaken thought that it is bad for the back to lie face down. All that is needed is to stretch the hip so that you are not pulled into an arch, but can comfortably straighten.

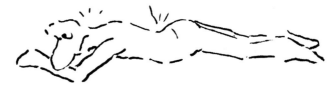

When the front of the hip has healthy resting length, you should be able to lie flat, both face up and face down, without tightness pulling you into painful arching.

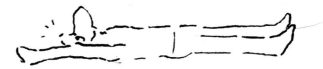

What to do for a tight hip

- The standing lunge is a combination hip stretch and leg strengthener. It also retrains how to bend properly. You know that bending over wrong is hurtful to the back. Use the lunge instead. Stand with one foot in front, one in back. Keep the back foot straight, not turned out. Bend both knees, keeping body weight centered between both legs. Tip your hip under to reduce low back arch. Feel the stretch in front of the hip on the back leg. The lunge is described more in Part II, next, in the section on how to use abs during yoga.

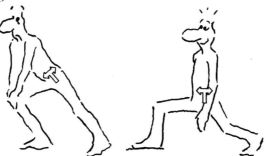

Don't lean forward, or tilt your hip forward in front (left). To stretch the front of your hip, tuck your hip with your weight distributed evenly between the front and back leg (right).

- When you stretch backward over an exercise ball, bed, pillow, or other object, check if the only way you stretch is to drape your arched back over the ball with your hip bent. This is counterproductive after spending most of their day with the hip bent. The purpose of the stretch is to lengthen and "unbend" the hip, not keep it bent.

- Place the ball (or other object) under your hip, not lower back, in order to stretch the front of your hip. If you feel pinching in your low back, tuck your hip to reduce the arch. Then you will stretch your hip, not just arch your back. Keeping the lower back arched and the front of the hip bent is not stretching your hip.

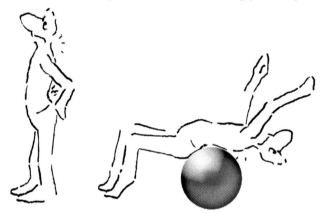

After standing all day with your lower back arched and hip bent (left), don't stretch with the same poor posture you are trying to prevent (right).

- When standing to stretch your quadriceps (thigh), tip your hip under to reduce the low back arch. You will feel the stretch move to the quadriceps and front muscles of your hip. Don't let your knee come forward. The point is to straighten your hip and stretch it back, not keep it bent forward. More on using your abdominal muscles for better quadriceps stretching is found on page 55.

- Watch for flexed posture by watching your clothing side seam or belt. Your side seam should not tilt forward between your waist and hip. Look at your belt line from the side view. If the belt tips down in front because you stand arched, tuck your hip back under. Don't push your hip forward.

- Lie on your back with your legs out straight. This is diagnostic for a tight hip. With healthy resting length of your front hip muscles, you can lie comfortably without your low back pulled up into an arch. A small normal space remains in the low back. It is not supposed to flatten to the floor. If you are too tight to lie flat without the low back overarching, you are too tight to stand without the same thing happening. The answer is not to stand and lie with the knees bent all the time but to stretch the front of the hip so that you can stand in healthy position without pain.

Part II
Ab Revolution™ Exercises for Functional Strengthening

This section is for using abdominal muscles
to maintain neutral spine during exercise,
from simple to challenging

Ab Revolution™ Exercises Work Your Abs
the Way You Need for Real Life

The conventional ab exercises you often see in gyms make you good at hunching forward. But your abs need to work isometrically (at one length without moving) a great deal of the time in real life, not bending forward. You need to exercise your abs the way they normally should work. This is called functional exercise. That means radically different exercises. The concepts and exercises follow in this section.

Ab revolution exercises work your abs in functional ways for postural control when you sit, stand, walk, run, carry packages, do exercise, and go out and have fun.

At first, many people cannot do these exercises for more than a few seconds. They don't have the ab strength and endurance to hold themselves straight. No wonder their posture sags so badly by the end of the day and their muscles ache. Gradually increase the time you hold your new healthy spine position with these exercises.

More important than how many repetitions you do, is understanding the concept of how abs work to change low back positioning. Use your abs to adjust your posture during the exercise and train your brain to transfer this body knowledge to all your daily activities. Doing repetitions and sets without that will not work your abs the way you need, and won't help your posture, your back, or your life. Breathe normally and fully when doing the isometric exercises; don't hold your breath. For the moving exercises, breathe in then breathe out during the effort of the movement.

Using abdominal muscles should not just be for doing exercise. Don't neglect using abs for standing and reaching properly all day every day. You will burn calories and get a free workout, and train functional ab use for posture, activities, back pain prevention, and good looks.

Real Athletes Use Abs

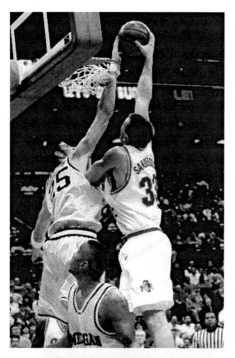

Both players in the photo at left show good use of abs to hold the spine in position while reaching upward to drive the dunk and power the block.

In the karate photo below, the black belts holding the board prevent overarching by using their abs. The force of the punch is not levered onto their low back. The white belt has not learned this yet. Note how he incorrectly uses an arch to draw back the punching arm.

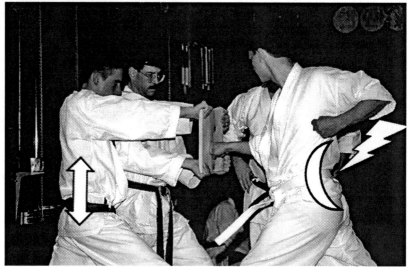

How to Use Abs When Doing "Non Ab" Exercises

Letting the lower spine overarch while lifting weight overhead compresses the lower spine and shifts the downward force of the weight to the joints of your spine instead of the core muscles. Overarching the lower back may be done for several reasons. It may just be allowed to happen without knowing it can make problems. Someone may deliberately arch, mistakenly thinking it should be done or that it looks good. It is also done because can make the lift easier because it shifts some of the weight off the muscles and onto the lower back. That is why it is hard on the lower back. For extreme weight, it may be the only way to get the weight lifted. For lifting for exercise and health, practice neutral spine instead and get the benefits of lifting in a healthier way.

Overhead press
Use your abdominal muscles to tuck your hips enough to reduce the large arch back to neutral spine. Sometimes you use abs to make a small adjustment, other times a larger one.

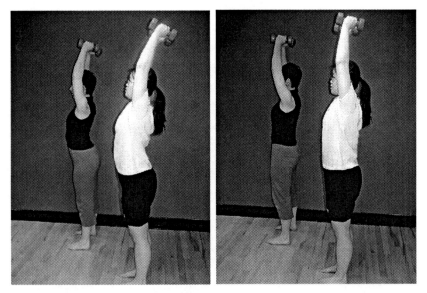

Left: Bad posture, arching the low back to lift the dumbbells.
Right: Same exercise using abdominal muscles to reduce the hyperlordosis back to neutral spine.

Triceps curls

Notice if you allow hyperlordosis to hold and lower the weight when doing overhead triceps curls. The lower back bears the weight instead of the torso and arm muscles. Arm exercise is diminished. You also miss the free abdominal workout you would get if you used your abdominal muscles to maintain healthier spine position.

Tuck the hip to make the line from the top of the leg to the middle of the crest of the hip vertical. If you were leaning the upper body back, pull forward to straight position.

By returning to neutral spine, you shift the weight of your upper body, plus the weights, off your lower spine. You will feel the effort shift to your core muscles.

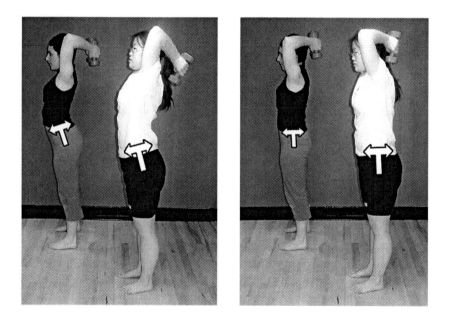

Left: Bad posture for triceps curls, overarching the low back.
Abdominal muscles are not in use. The beltline tips down in front.
The side seam from the top of the leg to middle hip crest tilts forward.
Right: Same exercise with abs in use to
reduce the hyperlordotic arch back to neutral spine.

Yoga

Yoga won't automatically "give" you good posture. Consciously use your muscles to move you into healthy spine position when practicing poses.

Some styles of yoga teach to deliberately stand in arched position. Letting the spine sag into lordosis does not use the abs and is hard on the back.

Instead, use your abdominal muscles to tuck your hip and reduce the arched posture to use neutral spine for poses such as warrior, tree of life, and many others, to increase core muscle exercise and prevent compression on the lower spine. You will also get a better leg stretch in many poses without over arching.

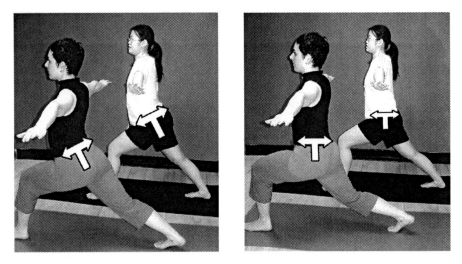

Left: Bad posture during Warrior series. Lower back overly-arched. Abdominal muscles not in use. The beltline tips down in front. The side seam from the bump at the top of the leg bone (greater trochanter) to the center of the hip tilts forward.
Right: Same pose done properly with abs in use to reduce the hyperlordotic arch back to neutral spine and control posture. More stretch in hip and leg.

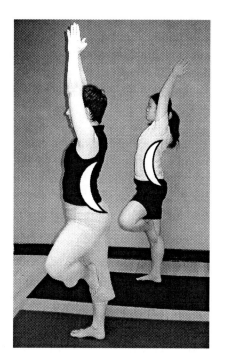 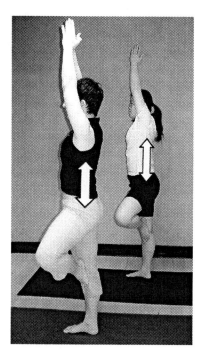

Left: Bad posture for Tree of Life pose.
Lower back overly-arched. Abs not in use.
Right: Same pose done with abs in use to reduce the hyperlordotic arch
and control spine positioning. Better stretch in hip and shoulder.

Allowing the lower spine to sag under your weight into compressive hyperlordosis during some poses is different from beneficial back extension which can be done as part of other poses, explained more on pages 99 and 100. In lying down extension exercise, your back muscles are pulling you upward, which unloads the discs, rather than compressing downward on the spine as happens in hyperlordosis. When lying down, there isn't the vertical (axial) spine compression from your upper body, as in standing.

In lying down back extension stretches, such as cobra and upfacing dog, check to see if you hang body weight on your lower spine joints and only extend backward from the area that most easily bends backward. Instead, use abdominal muscles to take weight off the lower spine and adjust the pose to spread the stretch over the length of the spine, particularly the upper spine. The lower spine is already good at bending backward. It usually does not need more hyperlordotic effort. However, the upper spine is often kept rounded forward in modern life. It needs the beneficial stretch the other way. Using the stretches in healthy ways can change a painful yoga routine to healthier practice.

For standing back extension stretches, such as crescent moon where you stand with both arms overhead and lean arms and upper body far backward, spread the backward stretch to the upper spine where it is needed, as above, and use abdominal muscles to support the extension to keep weight off the lower spine, explained more on pages 101 and 102.

Walking and Running
A common time to feel pain occurring from hyperlordosis is after walking or running. A small natural inward curve in the lower back functions as a spring for shock absorption, and keeps forces distributed evenly on your discs. When you maintain neutral spine, you will have the small inward curve. Exaggerating the curve allows body weight to grind down on the low back and decreases natural shock absorption. If you feel you must lean over or sit to relive discomfort when walking or running, check for neutral spine.

Archery
Archery is an activity where using abs saves more than your back. If you over arch the spine when drawing a bow, your chest will protrude outward into the line of the bowstring. You can painfully "twang" your breast with the bowstring. Tuck your chest and hip as if starting a crunch to straighten up. Don't curl forward. Hold good straight posture to keep your chest out of the line of the bowstring.

Target Practice
One of many techniques in target shooting is to "lock out" a stance to the end range of the joints to make the stance steadier, including a hyperlordotic lean-back of the upper body. In addition to bearing the body weight, the joints receive the impact of the firing. You can be steady in neutral spine. Use your abdominal muscles to keep you standing upright, not arched or leaning back. You will get steady shot and a free abdominal muscle workout.

How to Use The Ab Revolution™ for Stretching Your Legs

The anterior hip and quadriceps stretch is a common stretch where you can lose the intended stretch and add to back pain by arching. The arching is not caused by pulling the leg back but by allowing your hip to tilt forward in front. You can control whether you tilt or not. Try this:

- Stand on one leg and arch your back while you hold your other foot behind you. You won't feel much stretch in your thigh.

- Straighten your torso, tucking your hip as if starting to do a crunch. Drop your bent knee to point downward and push your foot away into your hand. Don't pull your foot in. Feel the stretch move to your thigh.

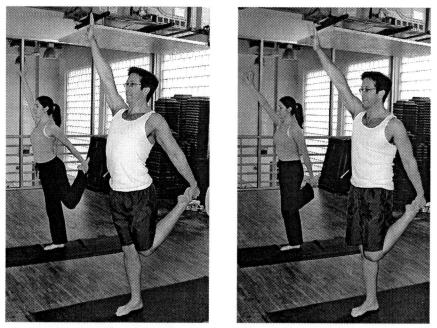

Left: Allowing the low back to arch. There is little stretch on the hip and thigh. Right: Same stretch using abdominal muscles to straighten spine position to neutral spine and increase leg stretch.

How to Use Abs for Stretching Your Arms

Check to see if you arch your lower back and lean back when stretching your arms. Arching adds to mysterious low back pain, and reduces the stretch in the shoulder. The following shows how to use your abdominal muscles to keep the healthy position you need to stretch your arms and shoulder more effectively. Try this:

- Stand up with arms high overhead and see if you allow your back to arch and ribs lift upward.

- With arms still overhead, flex your trunk as if starting a "crunch" to tuck the hip and spine position to neutral. Keep your elbow lifted to the ceiling. Don't bend your neck and head forward. Keep straight. Feel the stretch move to your shoulder and triceps.

- If you like to stretch the upper back at the same time, use supported back extension, pages 101 and 102.

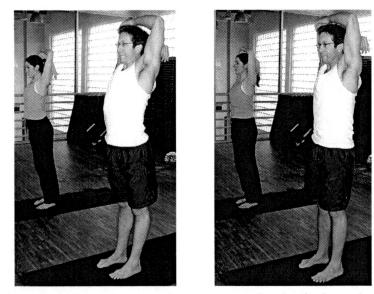

Left: Bad position when stretching arms overhead. The lower back is arched, with less stretch at the shoulder. Right: Same stretch using abdominal muscles to stop overarching and increase shoulder stretch.

Isometric Abs with Hand Weights

_____

"Isometric Abs" is a fun exercise to work your abs and learn to use them to hold healthy spine position against overhead resistance. "Isometric Abs" teaches you to feel when you are substituting arching your back for motion of the shoulder. This exercise also improves shoulder range of motion and function when lifting.

"Isometric abs" using body weight

- Lie on your back with your knees bent and feet on the floor. Put your hand on the floor under the arch of your lower back. Arch your back up and away from your hand, lifting your ribs high, so you know what arching the lower back feels like.

- To feel how to use abs to reduce the low back arch and control spine position, press your lower back down against your hand. Don't lift your hips, just use your abs. You will feel your abdominal muscles working right under the skin.

- Put your other arm overhead just off the floor, biceps by your ear. Did your back arch off your hand again? Press it back down.

- Now put both hands overhead, just an inch off the floor, biceps near your ears. Contract your abs to hold your torso straight without allowing your back to arch and lift far from the floor.

- Try the entire exercise again with both legs straight on the floor, not bent at the knee. If it is not comfortable or possible, the front of your hip may be too tight. Tight anterior hip is a common problem in lordosis. Tightness is easily solved by stretching the muscles in the front of the hip. See the end of Part I, pages 44-46. It explains why the tight hip adds to the problem of hyperlordosis, and tells how to stretch your hip to be able to walk, move, and even lie down comfortably with neutral spine.

Using hand weights
The Isometric Abs exercise using weights is excellent to develop abdominal muscles while learning how to use your abs to control your spine when lifting overhead.

- Lie on your back, holding dumbbells in each hand, arms by ears overhead, about an inch from the floor. Keep your elbows slightly bent.

- Don't let your ribs come up or your back arch. Press your low back downward to the floor. Don't strain. You will feel the weight shift off the low back and shoulder joints, and onto your abdominal muscles.

Your abdominal muscles work hard on this one to control your posture against the weight. Holding the weights also works your arms and latissimus dorsi muscles along the sides of your back. You get several exercises for the price of one, and work your body the way you need for real life movement.

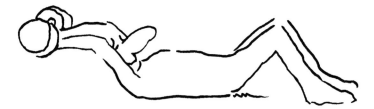

Use abdominal muscles to hold your spine in position without letting the weights pull your lower spine into overarching.

Moving with hand weights
- Raise and lower the dumbbells about an inch as many times as you can without touching the floor. Use abs to keep your lower back from rising off the floor at any time, particularly when lowering the weights.

- Each time the weight lowers, your back will want to arch. Don't let it. This simulates all the daily life activities where you will either maintain healthy spine position with your muscles or allow your back to arch and shift the weight to the joints of your back.

To train real life positioning, straighten your legs
- While holding hand weights, extend your legs straight to simulate lifting weight overhead while standing. Use your abdominal muscles to press your low back down toward the floor so that your back is not pulled by the weights into an overly arched position. There will be a small space between your lower back and the floor, but not a large arch.

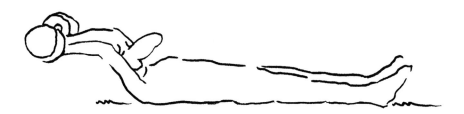

- If you are so tight that you cannot straighten your legs without your ribs lifting and your spine being pulled upward into a larger arch, you are too tight to stand straight and reach up without strain. You may need to stretch your front hip muscles (hip flexors) so that you can straighten your legs with healthy spine positioning when standing. Keeping the knees bent all the time does not solve the problem, it, perpetuates the source of the problem. Try the hip stretches on page 45. If your shoulders are uncomfortable, try the pectoral stretches on page 20.

But shouldn't you keep knees bent?
It is commonly taught that you must keep your knees and hips bent to "protect your back" and "keep your back from arching" and "to put your back into proper position" when doing ab and core exercise. However, your own abdominal muscles should position your back. By keeping knees bent, you never learn to use your muscles the way you need when standing up. You cannot walk or move properly in real life with knees and hips bent that much. Yet many people keep their hip bent all the time when standing, then exercise that way. Bending knees feeds a negative cycle of tight hip, bent hip, pain, and, ironically, an arched back just to stand up straight. The hip gets so tight that they need a pillow under their knees to sleep. What they need is to stretch the front of their hip so their hip and legs can extend enough for them to just stand up straight. Then they will no longer need the pillow.

Carry-over to real life

Think of the many exercises and daily life activities that involve lifting weight overhead—where you should stand without arching, as you have practiced in the "Isometric Abs" exercise. If you allow your back to arch, the force of the weight presses down on your low back. When you do standing weight lifting, and activities around the house like putting away laundry and groceries, remember to control your spine position with what you learned from the lying-down training exercise.

The Ab Revolution teaches you to understand how your muscles can move your spine out of unhealthy position to stop back pain, and how to retrain yourself to easily use safe, effective movement all the time so your back does not hurt in the first place.

Spine positioning does not come from bending your knees. If you use your abs for posture adjustment during all your standing movements, the isometric ab exercise will not only work your abs for the moment, but all day when you need it—standing up.

Ab Revolution™ Planks and Pushups

Holding a pushup position, without letting the low back sag or your behind hike upward, is a major way to train how to hold your back from sagging in unhealthy position under the pull of gravity when standing.

Pushups and planks (holding a pushup position) are often cited as good core muscle exercise. But, when they are done allowing the low back to arch, your weight rests on your vertebrae, not your "core" muscles. Letting the lower back arch is a missed opportunity to strengthen your core and is hard on your back. Don't let your back arch and you will train core stability and upper and lower body strength.

Even if you cannot do pushups, just holding a pushup position (plank), with straight positioning is a quick, effective exercise for most of your body, including the important weak link of wrists and arms.

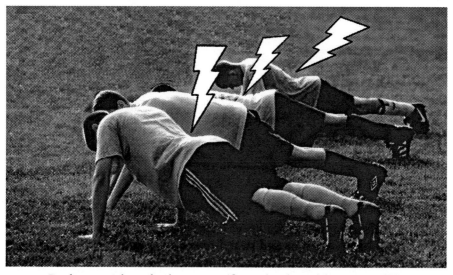

Pushups with arched posture (first, third, and last on right).
Abdominal muscles are not in use. The weight of the body
"hammocks" on the lower back joints (facets) and soft tissue.

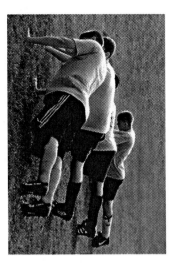

Turning the photo sideways shows how the first, third, and fourth boy would look standing up – overly arched, bad posture, head hanging, and lack of use of abs and other muscles.

Check to make sure you do not allow your spine to sag during pushups or when standing up.

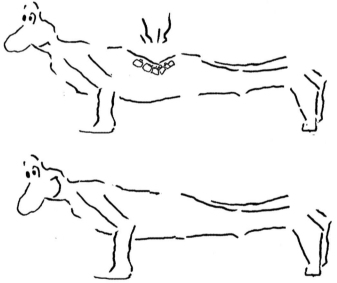

Upper drawing shows the lower back folding into a painful arch.
Instead, tuck your hips and straighten your back (lower drawing).
You will immediately feel your ab muscles in use.
The more you tuck to straighten, the more you use abs.

Don't tuck so much that you hunch your back or hike your hips in the air. Use abs to hold you straight, and you will save your back and change the pushup into an abdominal and core exercise that transfers knowledge of using abs to real life.

Holding the pushup position (plank)
- Hold the pushup position as long as you can. Tuck your hip to take the arch out of your back and straighten your torso. You will feel an immediate shift of the work to your abdominal muscles. Don't let your body droop down, or hike your hips up in the air. Hold your head up. Be straight as a plank. Photo below.

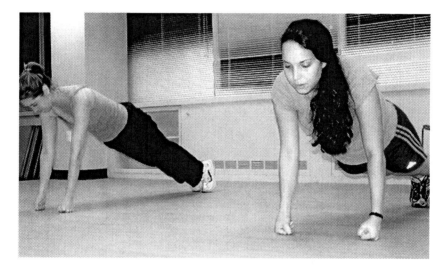

- Keep your elbows slightly bent; don't lock them straight. If your arms are too weak to hold you, you need to strengthen them, not ruin your elbow joints. Keep your weight on your entire hand; don't just mash your wrists.

- Vary hand positioning to strengthen hands.

Is your torso or neck wobbling and sagging after only a few seconds? These are the same posture muscles you need to stand properly without sagging. If you cannot hold up your own body weight, no wonder your back hurts at the end of the day. Work to increase the time you can hold your posture without sagging. If you lift weights to strengthen your back, remember that the most important weight to be able to lift is your own body.

If you cannot figure how to tuck your hips under you, stand up again and relearn the posture exercises in Part I on how to use your abs to control your posture when standing, on pages 15 and 28.

Planks lifting arms and legs

- Hold the pushup position as long as you can and lift one leg straight up in back without arching your back.

- Hold the pushup position and lift one leg in back and the opposite arm straight out in front. Don't let your body turn to the side. Stay level.

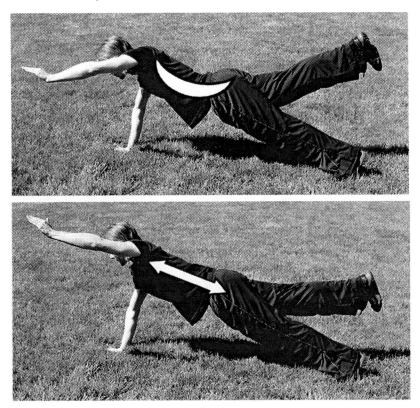

Top: Don't let your lower back sag into an arch.
Bottom: Tuck your hip and straighten your lower back.
Raise your arm level with your body. Keep your head up.

- Hold a pushup position on your elbows. Keep your hips tucked, back straight, and head up. Don't let your body sag toward the floor. Holding straight is just learning how to hold up your own body weight.

- Put your feet up on a bench or ledge or against a wall, photo below. Hold the pushup position without sagging. Keep your body straight as a plank.

- Use a low ledge to work abs more, and a higher one to work arms more.

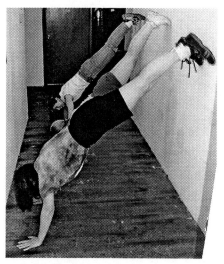

First from left is holding hip bent and hiked in the air.
Second and third are flatter and straighter.

Wheelbarrows
- The wheelbarrow can be a fun partner exercise. The first partner holds a plank, not allowing the lower back to sag. The second partner picks up the first partner's legs at the ankles.

- The second partner walks forward and to the sides in any direction holding the first partner's ankles while the first partner must walk on hands, maintaining neutral spine using abs.

- Advanced wheelbarrows can be done with both partners in plank and the first partner's feet on the second's shoulders. For more fun, add more partners to the wheelbarrow "train."

Hold the plank to lift weights
- Hold the pushup position on one arm and lift a hand weight from the floor to your chest with the other (like rowing), keeping straight body position. Try curls and other lifts.

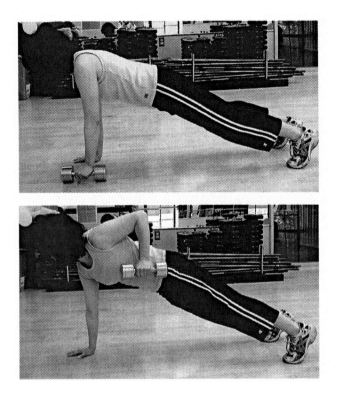

Reverse pushups
- Lie face down with hands on the floor and elbows bent at your sides ready to push up. Tuck your hip as if starting a crunch.

- Lift your body straight up in a reverse pushup without letting your upper body rise first, not even a small amount.

- Don't arch or hike your behind up in the air. Stay flat.

- Lower to the floor holding your body just as straight. Keep breathing and repeat all you can.

Increase weight to increase strength while holding position
Add a weight during pushups. Increased resistance increases strength and adds postural challenge. Start with a knapsack or other light weight.

Work up to holding more weight on your back—carefully—while keeping healthy spine position. Don't let your lower back sag under the weight. Use this exercise to learn to keep your back safe.

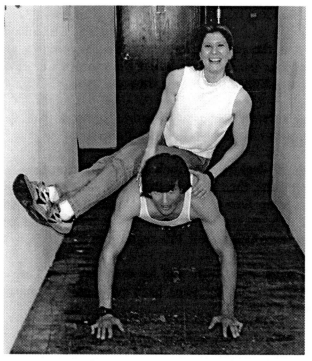

Adding extra weight means using more effort in abdominal and core muscles to keep your back in healthy position.

Walking and jumping pushups (spiders)
To increase strength, balance, power, and posture control, try these fun effective walking and jumping planks:

- "Walk" around in the pushup position like a flat spider. Tuck your hips under as if starting a crunch to keep your back straight. Walk sideways, forward, backward, and around. Walk quickly and slowly. Maintain the same posture you would want if you were standing up. Stay straight. Keep your head up.

- Jump in the pushup position like a flat jumping spider. Don't allow your back to arch under the momentum of landing. Use good shock absorption with arms and legs.

- Jump sideways across the room. Jump to the next piece of furniture or exercise equipment. Jump to say hello to someone.

- Jump 90 degrees with each jump to face each direction. Start facing front, then jump to the left, back, right, then front again. Then jump four times back the other way–from front to right, back, left, to the front again. Have fun. Work up to full half turns, eventually to full 360-degree jumps.

"Spiders" work torso, arm, and leg muscles hard. They are effective and safe if you protect your back with good posture and shock absorption.

Challenge moves
As you advance, work to hold your body straight without support for the feet. These moves are sometimes called "The Flag." Experiment with varied leg placement.

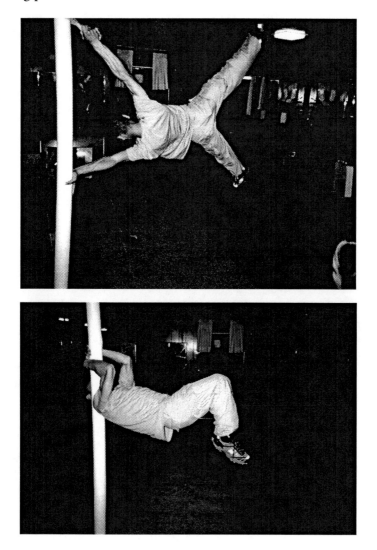

Using Oblique Abs to Control Core Positioning—Side Arm Standing

Check if you let your body slump to one side, or hike your shoulder or hip up when carrying things on one side. Sometimes people slouch to the side even when just standing. Side arm standing (side planks) work your oblique abdominal muscles. Train yourself to use your obliques to also hold your torso straight when standing and carrying loads.

Holding side pushup position (side plank)
- Hold the pushup position and turn to one side. Lift one arm and balance on the other arm, holding your body straight without drooping. Keep your elbow slightly bent; don't lock it straight. Save your elbow joint and get an arm workout. Keep your weight on your whole hand not just the heel of the hand, so that you don't compress your wrist. Hold as long as you can then switch sides and repeat.

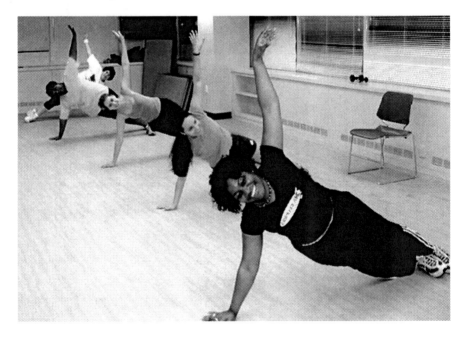

Use side planks to consciously train straight torso positioning
to transfer to use when standing.

- For variation, prop on one elbow. Progress to putting your feet up on a ledge or bench, or up against the wall. Use the free arm to lift a hand weight up and down in various arm lifts, presses, and curls.

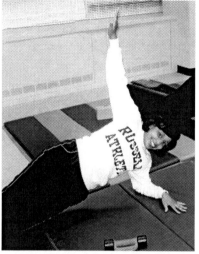

- In the side position, raise your top leg and hold.

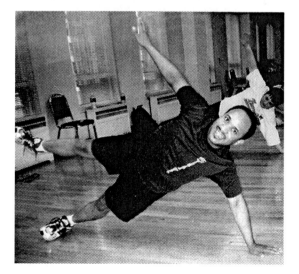

- For variation, move the top leg forward and hold it out in front as long as you can. Then try stretching the raised leg behind you, both straight-leg, and bending the knee.

Moving in the side arm position
- Hold the side arm position and raise and lower your top leg from the floor as many times as you can, maintaining straight torso posture.

- Hold the side arm position and dip your hip almost to the floor and raise up as many times as you can.

- Do the same dip holding your top leg off the floor.

- Hold a side arm position and continuously switch arms, turning side to side maintaining straight positioning.

Benefit to wrists
The wrist is one of the three major sites of osteoporosis. Weight bearing exercise improves arm bone density and strength, two more benefits of Ab Revolution exercises. To prevent wrist pain, keep your weight distributed on your entire hand not just the heel of the hand. Press using the muscles of your hands and fingers, so that you do not compress your wrist backward. Many cases of wrist pain, attributed to carpal tunnel syndrome, are just weak wrists that are compressed under body weight during movement without use of the surrounding muscles.

Check when you type, drive, prepare food, and during other daily activities that you are not angling the wrists backward. There is no need to hold the wrist straight or splint it. Movement is crucial for all joint health. Use hand strength when using your hands, don't just let all the weight fall backward or twist on the wrist joints. Using arms and hand muscles will relieve wrist pain the same way that using torso muscles and positioning relieves the pressure on the low back. Using hand and arm muscles will also strengthen your hands and wrists so that your wrists are no longer squashed under everyday activity.

More Challenging Ab Revolution Moves for Oblique Abdominal Muscles

- Hold a regular facedown pushup position. Lift 1 leg 90 degrees to the side with toes forward, as if swinging it over a bicycle. Keep your leg straight and parallel to the floor, not drooping down. Sometimes this exercise is called "The Peeing Dog" for the position of the leg straight up and out to the side.

- Keep your body flat, not turned to the side. Don't let your lower back sag down. Don't stick your behind up. Hold good position as long as you can, then switch legs. Work up to switching legs by jumping from leg to leg, instead of putting one down before lifting the other.

- Try pushups while holding the leg straight out to the side.

- When you can hold your leg out straight to the side, add lifting the opposite arm.

- Jump to change the lifted arm and leg.

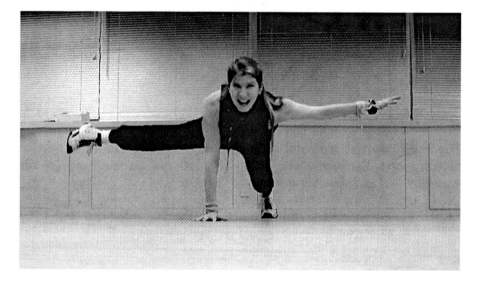

Using Abs, Not Hands, to Reposition the Spine for Leg Lifts

Leg lifts may sometimes be taught with the instruction that hands under the hip "keep the back from arching." However, using hands prevents you from using your own abdominal muscles to keep your back from arching.

By not taking the arch out of your back with your own abdominal muscles, leg lifts don't work your abdominal muscles, but shift more of the exercise to the muscles that lift your leg, called hip flexors. Hip flexors are usually strong and tight to begin with, from sitting and overuse in conventional exercises. Tight hip flexors create many problems, including back pain and change in ability to move in healthy ways. Leg lifts are not a functional exercise for most things. Most people do not need to practice bending from the hip. They are already too tight and bent.

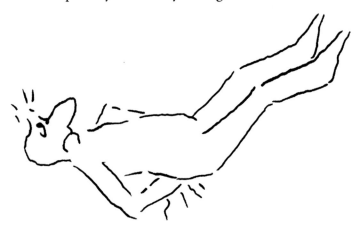

For ballet, martial arts, and rock climbing, leg lifts can help practice certain moves. For people who do leg lifts, use your abs, not hands, to tilt your hips and maintain torso posture. Try this:

- Lie on your back with legs out straight. Put one hand under the small of your lower back, and feel the natural space.

- To learn what arching feels like, increase the arch by lifting your ribs so that your back lifts off your hand. In this arched position, lift your legs just an inch or two above the floor. You will feel the weight of your legs pulling your back into more of an arch, pinching and straining your lower back. (Don't do this if you have back pain.) This is how many people do leg lifts. It can be injurious and does not use abs.

- To fix the arching problem, put your legs back down and press your lower back against your hand, using your abs to flatten the arch. If your hips are tight, you may feel your thighs pull upward. Try not to let them pull up. Holding them straight will retrain your muscles to know what it feels like to use abs to control torso posture.

- While keeping your abs in use to hold the spine straight, lift your legs just an inch or two above the floor. Don't let your back arch. You will feel your abs working. Don't let your back arch during any point of raising or lowering your legs.

Learn to use your abs, not your hands, to change the tilt of your torso and hips. You will learn to use your abdominal muscles to control your torso posture. You will protect your back, and get more abdominal exercise.

Hanging leg lifts
When you do leg lifts hanging from a bar or overhead support, don't allow your back to arch. Use abdominal muscles to straighten your body. When you lift your legs, don't just bend at the hip with your behind stuck out. First, curl your hips under you, doing a "reverse crunch" while hanging. Then, while maintaining the curled position of your torso, lift your legs. Keep your torso posture controlled with your abs as you lower your legs too, not allowing it to arch.

Back leg lifts
Exercising the muscles of the back as needed for life is important. One conventional back exercise is to bend over forward and lift weights. You already know this is what you should not do to pick up a package. It works the muscles but is harmful to the discs, over time. Instead, one good exercise for healthy and effective back muscle strengthening is back extension. Some extension exercises follow. More are shown in the chapter on Back Extension That Helps Reduce Back Pain, page 99.

Leg lifts to the back (lower back extension) contract and strengthen back muscles. Watch for the mistake of arching the back to lift the leg, not by lifting with the hip and leg muscles. Arching reduces involvement of the leg and back muscles, compresses the lower spine joints, and reinforces faulty movement patterns—to move your leg by arching your spine.

In the same way, watch for the same injurious body mechanics of arching when walking and running, instead of maintaining neutral spine and using muscles of the leg and hip to extend the leg.

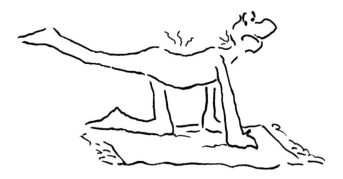

When lifting your leg to the back, don't arch your back to lift your leg. Tuck your hip under to bring your back to a straight position and use your leg, hip, and gluteal muscles to lift your leg. You will feel an immediate shift of work to your abs, and far more exercise for your back and leg. You may find you cannot lit your leg as high. That is because you were not previously lifting with your leg muscles, but lifting your leg by arching your back, pivoting on the spine joints. Now you will be getting real leg exercise, while getting built-in abdominal exercise.

Remember not to crane or pinch your neck backward. Use upper back muscles to hold your head and neck up with chin in, don't just bend your neck at an angle. Let your chest lift up to look forward without craning your neck and arching your lower back.

Whenever you do leg lifts, use Ab Revolution repositioning to get a better abdominal workout, and to learn how healthy posture feels when controlling your torso. Then transfer the knowledge of how to use good positioning to all your daily activities when standing.

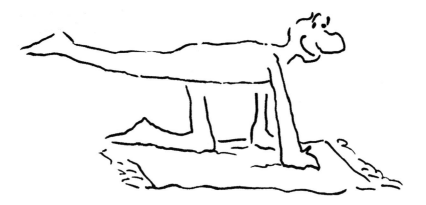

The "hands and knees position" gives little exercise and does not train you how to hold your body weight up against gravity. Instead of spending time on ineffective exercises, get off your knees. Hold a real pushup position. It will strengthen your arms and better strengthen your body in a functional way. Make sure to use abdominal muscles to tuck your hip under to straighten your spine, or you will get little core exercise. Then try lifting one leg, holding healthy straight position.

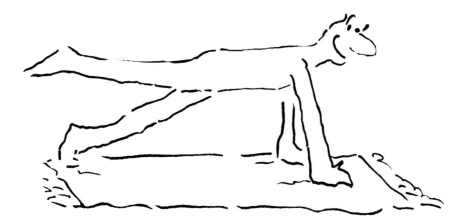

Using abdominal muscles to prevent your spine from sagging when lifting your leg while holding the "plank" will not only give you effective abdominal exercise, but retrain you how not to let your back arch when you extend your legs back to walk.

When you can hold a straight plank with one leg up, hold the straight plank position lifting one arm straight in front. Don't drop your head. Use your muscles to hold you as straight as if you were standing. Then try holding your arm out in front, while lifting the opposite leg up in back. Maintain straight spine position.

Chin-ups and pull-ups

Check if you stick out your behind and let your legs swing forward when doing chin-ups and pull-ups. Instead, use your abs to tip your hip under you into straight position, and keep your legs and body straight while raising and lowering.

To train oblique abs and front abdominal fibers lower along their length while doing pull-ups and chin-ups, use the hip tuck described above and in the section on leg lifts. Hang from the bar and take the arch out of your back by using your abs to curl your hips under you. Don't allow your body to swing forward or your back to arch as you pull up. Keep your torso positioning controlled as you lower down. Retrain away from the postural habit of doing pull-ups with the hip bent, ribs jutting forward, and the lower back arched. Holding straight positioning gives effective and functional use of abdominal muscles.

Ab Revolution™ Bands

Using bands or cable pulleys

- Use cable pulleys, or secure the middle of a stretchy band or tube at head height or above. Turn your back. Hold one end in each hand. Lift arms overhead, preventing your lower back posture from arching. Step away to increase tension on the band. Don't let your arms pull behind you or your back arch.

- Try arm movements that simulate your sport (pitching, rowing, basketball) or activities like washing hair, controlling torso posture with your abs. This exercise practices maintaining posture against gravity and loads of daily life. Bands are also fun to do with a partner.

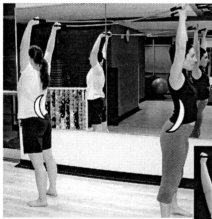

Bad posture.
Back arched.
Abs not in use.

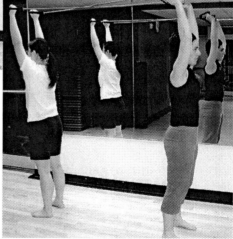

Using abs to
straighten posture
and increase exercise.

Ab Revolution™ Bands for Oblique Abdominal Training

This set of exercises trains you to use your oblique (side) abdominal muscles to hold your posture against resistance. You will strengthens your oblique abdominal muscles while learning how to hold your spine from slouching to the side when reaching and lifting overhead.

Not using abdominal muscles for arm tasks is a common contributor to shoulder pain. By not using your torso to power the move, you overload and over-rotate your shoulder. Over-rotation can occur in sports like swinging a tennis racquet, or in a high brace in kayaking, and in daily life. Reaching over the car seat for heavy items in the back seat without using supporting musculature frequently adds to rotator cuff injury.

Using bands and pulleys
- Use a stretchy band, tubing, pulleys, or even a pair of stretch pants to get started. Secure the middle at about shoulder height. Hold both ends and turn sideways.

- Move away to increase tension on the band.

- Maintain straight posture. Hold your torso stable against the sideways pull of the stretchy cord. Don't let the band pull you into bend sideways posture.

- Feel how to stabilize and straighten your body using your oblique abs.

- Swivel your body away from the resistance. Keep your knees bent and turn from your legs and hips, keeping your torso straight, not twisting from your waist.

- To progress, hold both arms overhead against your ears and repeat this exercise, always holding your body straight against the pull of the band.

Oblique ab exercise turning at various angles
- Hold the band at a strong tension and face various angles toward and away from the band. Practice moving your arms for common activities, retraining yourself to use abs first, before moving your arms. Try the motion of combing your hair (or washing your head, if you're bald), brushing teeth, hanging up clothes, writing on the board, underhand and side pitches, and anything else you need for daily life. Each time, instead of starting the move with your shoulder and arm, move your spine into straight position and feel the increase in use of the abdominal muscles first. Then, use the power of the torso (core) muscles to turn your body and power the arm movement.

Moving stabilization drills
- Walk around, side to side, and diagonally, keeping your body stable and straight against the changing pull of the band.

- Have a friend hold the other end of the band and pull you in odd directions while you practice torso stabilization. This simulates walking a dog, or carrying packages and a squirming baby while trying to get in the door.

- Swing a hula-hoop around your waist. Try it again, swinging it around your arms. Try swinging the hula hoop around one arm while moving against the resistance of the band held in the other hand.

Kettlebells and other heavy training devices are covered in the next section.

Ab Revolution—Throwing, Swinging, and Overhead Arm Activities

The exercises in this section teach how to use abs for speed and power while protecting your shoulder and lower back work during swinging and throwing arm movement overhead and around the body. When throwing and swinging, avoid the bad habit of arching the low back and flinging your arm. The fulcrum becomes the shoulder and lower back joints instead of the core and hip muscles. In baseball pitches and tennis serves, for example, by not positioning your torso first, you can overload your shoulder or elbow. Injury can eventually develop.

Using bands or cables
- Use cable pulleys, or secure the middle of a stretchy band or tubing at about shoulder height. Hold one end. Turn your back. Move away to increase tension on the band while standing straight. Don't allow the resistance to pull your back into an arch or pull your arm behind you. Feel how to stabilize and straighten your body and stand straight by using your abdominal muscles.

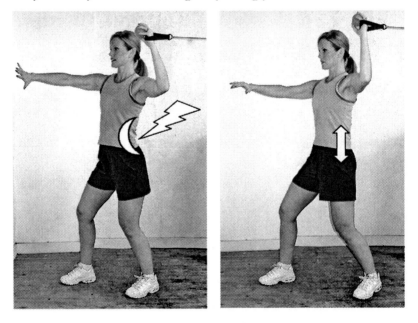

Left: Bad posture, back arched, abs not in use. Right: Abs in use to properly change spine posture and power the throw.

- Simulate throwing a ball with one arm. Push off your feet, turn your hip, and contract your abs so that your torso curls to neutral spine. Then swing the arm forward in a pitching/throwing action. Feel the pivot coming from your abs, not your shoulder.

Swinging a medicine ball, kettlebell, India Club, and heavy objects

Swinging heavy objects has long been done in many cultures. Objects may be a medicine ball on a rope, bowling pin shaped clubs (India clubs) that are thrown, juggled, and swung, bolos (to sling stones for hunting and target practice), stones with handles (many names from each culture that uses them, for example, chikairashi, kettlebells, yirevoy, chishi, and others), the Kwan-tao (General Kwan's heavy kung-fu ax), heavy poi chains, swinging dumbbells, and other heavy training objects.

Use your abdominal muscles to position the torso first to and stabilize the shoulder, then initiate action with your arm. Check if you allow your lower back to arch when swinging overhead, especially as the object swings behind you. Use abdominal muscles strongly to keep neutral spine.

Add balance and stability components

Do any of the Ab Revolution throwing and swinging exercises while standing on one foot. One foot training adds balance, strength, and stabilization training for your core, legs, and feet.

Ab Revolution™ on the Exercise Ball

The exercise ball is a large, inflated ball that you can use to exercise and stretch in many ways. It is called "Swiss Ball," "rehab ball," "therapy ball," "gym ball," "balance ball," "physio-roll," and any number of other trade names.

Because the ball is not flat, and rolls under you, there are claims of increased balance and stabilization during use. However, it is easy to sit or lie on the ball with little muscle use. There are claims that the ball makes you sit properly, or that you use more muscular effort to sit using the ball. Based on that assumption, expensive desk chairs are marketed with the ball as the sitting surface. However, you can sit on a ball with as poor posture and little effort as on most other surfaces.

Used properly, the exercise ball can be fun and effective, and use more body skills and muscles than doing the same exercise on a floor, chair, or bench. You do this by using muscles to deliberately to control posture. Used without understanding, the ball is just another device that does little, and reinforces the same poor habits as other exercises.

Crunches or reverse crunches done on a ball have all the same problems of postural impairment and lack of application to real life as crunches off the ball. Sitting on a ball (with both feet on the ground) and doing crunches on a ball are two of the least effective uses of the ball.

The ball can be put to better use with functional exercises that strengthen and train your core and other muscles to work the way you need for good posture, sports, and daily life. All the exercises that follow work your entire torso and back at the same time. Many strengthen arms and legs too. Try the following with safety and good judgment:

- Hold a pushup position with hands on the floor and the ball under your ankles. Tuck your hip to straighten spine position. Do not let your spine sag under your own weight.

- As you progress, do pushups with your feet up on the ball and your spine held straight. Keep your head up, not hanging down.

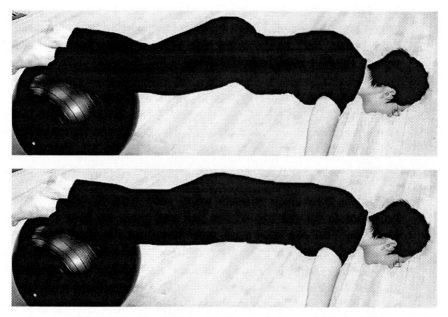

Top photo: Don't let your back arch or your behind hike up.
Bottom photo: Straighten your spine position to work your
abs and train healthier posture.

- While holding the pushup position with your feet on the ball, "walk" your hands back toward the ball until your chest is on the ball. Hold your legs straight out in space using back muscles.

- Turn over to lie with your shoulders on the ball, heels on the floor. Keep your legs and body straight. Don't arch or drape your back over the ball. Keep the same good posture as for healthy standing.

- Lie face up and "walk" your feet until the ball is under your behind, not letting your back arch or drape over the ball. Your upper body is held out in space by your abdominal muscles. Keep the ball under your behind, not your back. Hold as long as you can. Lift up one leg and hold as long as you can. Switch legs. Are you advanced? Lift both legs at once, lying flat and horizontal.

- Without using your arms, roll on the ball to lie on your side. Keep the side of your feet on the floor and the ball close to your hip. Hold straight posture as long as you can. For more, lift both arms over your head, biceps by ears. Advanced? Hold a weight in your hands. Roll to the other side without using your arms and repeat. Practice straight positioning.

- Roll onto your back without using arms. Step your feet away until the ball cradles your head and neck. Keep straight torso posture without sagging or arching. Hold. Lift one leg up straight and hold as long as you can out straight in the air. Switch legs and hold.

- Roll onto your chest without using your arms to turn you. Put both hands on the top of the ball and push up into a pushup position. You can start with your knees on the floor but don't raise the upper body by first arching at the lower back. Lift straight up. Don't let your back sag downward or hike up in the air. Hold as long as you can. To progress, do pushups with hands on the ball, holding spine straight without sagging. As you advance, roll to one side and balance on one arm at a time.

- Lie on your back on the floor, legs straight, with the ball under your ankles. Lift hips from the floor. Make sure to hold your body straight, don't let your neck bend under your body weight. Lift one leg from the ball. Hold. Repeat. Switch sides and repeat. Your back and leg muscles work strongly along with your abdominal muscles to do this exercise.

- Roll over to the pushup position with your feet on the ball and hands on the floor. Lift one leg up off the ball. Keep good posture without letting your back arch or hike up in the air. Hold as long as you can. Switch legs and hold. Photo next page.

- Hold the pushup position with one foot on the ball, the other lifted off the ball. Do pushups with one leg lifted and the hip tucked to straighten spinal position. Switch legs and repeat.

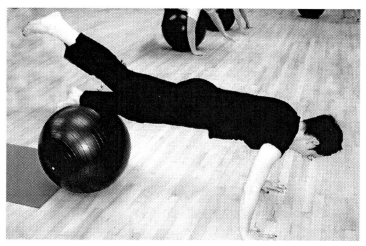

Lift one leg holding straight torso posture. Holding straight shifts body weight off the lower back and onto the abdominal muscles.
Then try pushups this way.

- Hold the pushup position with both feet on the ball and both hands on the floor. Turn your body all the way to one side, lifting one arm up straight to the sky to stand sideways on one arm with feet up on the ball. Hold straight body position. Hold as long as you can, then switch sides, keeping both feet on the ball.

- Hold a straight pushup position with both feet up on the ball and both hands on the floor. Lift one leg off the ball 90 degrees to the side with toes forward, and leg straight and parallel to the floor. This is the same "The Peeing Dog" position as page 73, but with one leg up on the ball. Then try it with the other arm lifted, holding all body segments straight and flat.

- Try "The Peeing Dog" as above, but with your hands on the ball, one foot on the floor, the other 90 degrees to the side. Then try it with the other arm lifted, holding all body segments straight and flat.

- Have fun making up more Ab Revolution moves on the ball.

Ab Revolution™ for Punching

For punching in martial arts and aerobic kickboxing classes, an arched lower spine posture generates injurious force on the lower spine, not only when punching but receiving a blow. Overarching is also an indication of reduced punching force, because core muscles are not driving the punching arm. The fulcrum of the punch becomes the lower back instead of the muscles of the abs, chest, and hip.

Training abdominal muscles for punching

- Stand near a wall. Stretch your arm forward in punching position. Don't hit the wall; just push the wall with your fist with your arm extended.

- Allow the push of your arm to arch your back. Lean the upper body backward and tilt the hip forward in front. Push increasingly hard. You may feel pressure or a familiar ache in your lower back. (Don't do this if you have back pain.)

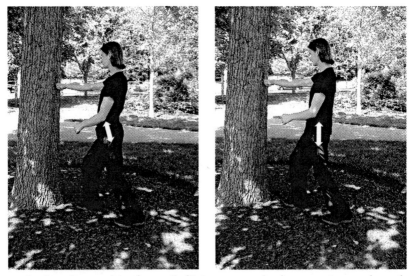

Tilting the hip forward in front (left) increases the lower spine arch and injurious pressure. It reduces power of the punch. Instead, tuck the hip to straighten the hip from leg to center hipbone (right). Hold upper body upright. Lower back pressure stops and punching power increases.

- Correct your spine position with your abs, as if beginning a crunch but not curling your neck forward. Tuck the hip under. Your hip shifts from stuck out in back to straight from the top of the leg bone to the middle of the crest of the hip. You should feel lower back pain disappear and a new strength in your punching arm.

- Whenever you punch, use the new neutral spine position, learned above. Don't allow your back to arch at any point. Don't hunch or round forward. Rounding puts your chin closer for your opponent to hit.

- Punching should not initiate from the arm or shoulder, but from the lower body. First, tip your hip under to reduce arching. Push off your feet, turn your hips, exhale, and keep the push coming from your abs to push your torso and arm forward. Don't arch your lower back.

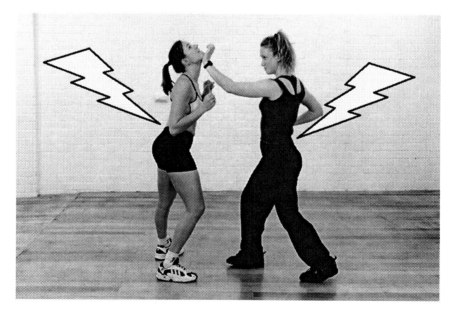

In both puncher and receiver, the overarched spine transmits force to the lower back and reduces ability to generate power.

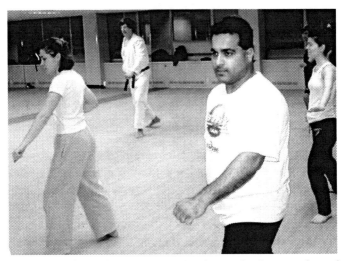

Can you spot the students not using abs in the karate class above?
(First on the left to a small degree and on right to a higher degree.)
They are overarching the spine, pressuring the lower back
and reducing punching power.

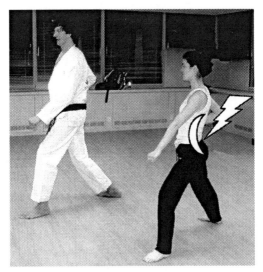

Teacher (left) is holding neutral spine.
Student (right) leans the upper body backward and tips the hip forward,
increasing injurious hyperlordotic arch. Student is also hyperextending
the elbow, not good for the elbow joint or the punch.

Ab Revolution punching using bands

- Use a stretchy band, rubber tubing, or cable pulleys, with the middle secured around anything solid at shoulder height or above. Turn your back, holding each end of the cord.

- Move far enough away to increase effort needed.

- Keep both arms in front of you. Don't let the resistance pull your arms behind you.

- Feel how to straighten your torso and hold neutral spine using your abdominal muscles. Maintain neutral spine position, not pulled backward or leaning forward.

- Contract your abs first before pushing with your arm. Push off your feet and legs, turn your hip into the punch, then using your abdomen as the fulcrum lever your arm forward into a powerful punch. Breathe out as you punch.

- Punching with bands can be done by looping your band around something behind you, or back-to-back with a partner holding their band looped around yours.

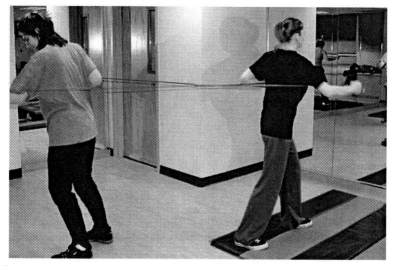

Photo shows improperly leaning forward. Stand upright against the pull of the bands, not pulled backward or leaning forward.

Using Abs for Pushing

All the abdominal muscles come into use for pushing things (front, oblique, and transversus) against heavy resistance. The following pushing exercise trains healthy, strong torso and back posture during pushing and slow powerful moves.

- Stand with both hands against a wall. Let your back arch. Begin pushing the wall with your hands, without bending your elbows. Allow the push of your arm to arch your back. Push increasingly hard. You will feel pressure, maybe the familiar ache in your lower back. (Don't do this if you have back pain.)

- Fix your spine position with your abs, as if beginning a crunch but not bending your neck or upper body. Tuck your hip under you, so your body is in a slight curl. You should feel the back pain disappear and a new strength.

- Breathe in, tuck your hips, press off your feet, use your hips and abdomen as the fulcrum, and breathe out as you lever your upper body forward in powerful pushing action.

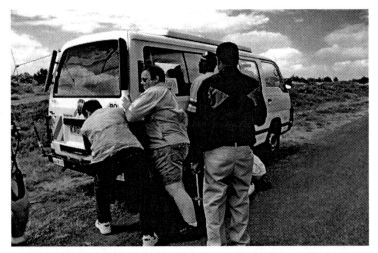

Prevent arching when pushing heavy objects. You will prevent lower back pain and generate more pushing force.

Ab Revolution™ for Kicking

In exercise and martial arts classes, check for allowing the lower back to arch when kicking to the side and back. The fulcrum of the kick becomes the lower back joints instead of the muscles of the abdomen and hip. The following kicking exercises train your abs while learning safe torso and back posture during kicking and leg movement in many sports from martial arts, to soccer, to swimming.

Train abs for kicking

- Stand sideways to a wall at a distance to swing a side kick. Put the bottom of your foot against the wall as if you just finished a side kick.

- Let your back arch. Begin pushing the wall with your foot without allowing your knee to give way. You may feel pressure; maybe the familiar ache in your lower back that you get from days (years) of bad posture habits. (Don't do this if you have back pain.)

- Fix your posture by using your abs as if beginning a crunch, but not bending your upper body forward. Straighten your back out of the arch. You should feel the back pain disappear and a new strength in your kicking leg. Do not curl the hip under, which increases pressure on the lower back discs, another kind of injury.

- With the new supported posture, practice your side kick. Don't allow your back to arch at any point in your kick. Maintain your slightly tucked posture. Don't hunch or round your back. Rounding is bad for your back and puts your chin closer to your opponent to hit.

- Try the same technique for a back kick. Stand facing away from a wall. Put the bottom of your foot against the wall. Feel the difference between letting your back arch, and tucking enough to straighten your back without rounding it.

Train abs for front kicking using bands
The following exercises can be done by using a cable pulley, using a band looped around something behind you at about hip height or below, or back to back with a partner holding their band looped around yours.

- Secure the band or cable handle around one leg and turn your back to the resistance of the band.

- Step away to put tension on the band. Don't let the pull of the band pull your back into an arch. Feel how to stabilize and straighten your body using abs to stand up straight.

- Contract your abs first. Push off your standing leg. Do not curl your upper body forward. Using your abdomen as the fulcrum, breathe out as you lever your leg forward into a powerful kick. Keep your standing heel down when you kick. Don't round your back forward to throw the kick. Hold straight.

Train abs for side and back kicking using bands
- Secure one end of the band or tubing handle around one leg. Turn to the side against the resistance of the band. Use your abs to hold your posture from arching during the kick.

- Try the same technique for a back kick. Stand facing wherever you have tied one end of the band. Secure the other end to your foot and kick backward. If you have tied both ends of the band to something secure (or are holding the ends) push your foot backward against the middle of the band. Feel the difference between letting your back arch when you kick backward, and tucking enough to straighten your back without rounding it.

What About Abdominal Twists?

An exercise commonly done for abs is to put a bar across the shoulders, and twist from side to side. The idea is that torso muscles would get exercise by decelerating the swinging weight. Check to see if you do this exercise in a way that does not work the abs, but over-twists the back.

Along with the bent forward neck posture from putting a bar across the shoulder, a big problem comes from stopping the momentum of the weight at the end of each rotation using vertebral joints, not abdominal muscles. The resulting rotational force (torque) on the spine can eventually strain soft tissue, fray discs, and overstretch the tendons that hold muscles on bones, and ligaments that hold your bones together.

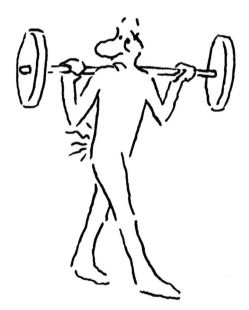

For activities that require body knowledge of how to decelerate a swinging pivot, such as swinging a bat or racquet, swinging limbs in martial arts, for dancing, or rodeo activities, learn to use your core muscles. Instead of allowing the rotation to swing your body to the limit that your spine twists, stop the momentum by using your abdominal and torso muscles to decelerate the weight through muscular effort.

If all you want is a pivoting ab exercise to work your abs, use cable pulleys or a stretchy tube or band and pivot away from it. There will be no momentum continuing the motion past the point where you pull the band. Use movements that are like real daily life activities to make it functional exercise. Practice throws, punches, serves, paddling motions, swings, and anything else you need to train for better real life motion.

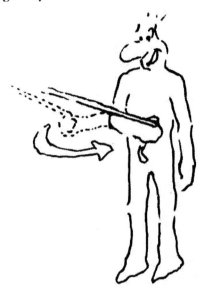

The ab study mentioned in the beginning of this book rated stretchy tubing low on the ranking of ab exercises that produce ab muscle activation. One reason is that they used the tubing while bending forward, rather than in real-life movements. Another possibility is not using enough resistance on the band. To get a useful effective exercise, use a good, thick band, step away to increase tension while holding good spine and body positioning, and go for the fun of the work.

How Many, How Often?

_____

How many of each exercise should you do?
Start by doing as many of each exercise as you can in healthy position. Use that as your base number. Work up to more.

Many easier ones, or fewer harder ones?
Regularly lift a weight that is so heavy that you can only lift it a few times builds strength. Lifting a lighter weight for a long time builds endurance. You need both for carrying things, for most daily activities, and just getting through the day with healthy posture, without a tired, achy back. For many people, their own body weight is so heavy relative to their ability that it provides enough resistance to build strength, for example pushups, handstands, and pull-ups. As you strengthen, you can do more repetitions, then gradually add external weight, building both strength and endurance.

How fast or slow?
Working muscles slowly gets them good at slow movement. That is good for carrying things and pushing cars (if you also trained to be strong enough). It will not make you able to do fast movements needed for real life activities like throwing, punching, blocking punches, catching falling objects or children, swinging a bat or racquet, or anything where you need your strength quickly. Practice exercises both quickly and slowly to maximize real life abilities. When going slowly with weights, don't tighten your joints or push them past their range. When going quickly, don't bang your joints around; use muscular control to avoid injury. Remember the purpose – healthier real life that is fun, not grunting your way through an artificial exercise.

When to do Ab Revolution exercises?
Use all the back-saving, arch-preventing core positioning exercises in this book all the time when you are standing, going about your normal day, and when doing exercise. Use your abdominal muscles to fix your spine positioning and support your body weight and the weight of what you carry for a free workout all the time.

"Ab-Only" Exercises Are Not Good

There are two main problems with doing conventional forward-bending abdominal muscle exercise programs or attending "abs" classes with the intention to reduce back pain or injury.

Abdominal muscles and back muscles are different muscles. Doing conventional abdominal muscle exercise does not work your back muscles any more than walking makes your arms strong. To strengthen your back, you have to work your back muscles with exercises that contract them. These are introduced in the pages that follow. It is true that using abdominal muscles to reposition your spine out of an unhealthy arch stops the pain from overarching, and there is a small effect on the back muscles called co-contraction. However, saying that forward-bending abdominal exercise strengthens your back muscles is not true.

Doing conventional ab exercises, which contract your abs to round you forward adds to "round-shoulders" upper crossed syndrome, and other upper and lower back pain. The forward-rounding posture puts unhealthy compression on discs, vertebrae, and nerves that exit the vertebrae. Forward slouching, from sitting rounded and exercising rounded, overstretches your back muscles and slowly pressures discs to bulge outward. Keeping your back muscles, or any muscles, lengthened by poor posture weakens them.

Rounding forward is a poor posture that people are usually good at, and spend a large portion of the day doing. A common approach is to do conventional abdominal exercises by bending forward, then turn over to do a few back extension exercises. Doing back extensions will not undo a day of unhealthy forward rounding. A better approach is to use the Ab Revolution exercises in this book to exercise the back and abdominal muscles at the same time, and in functional ways. Then add to back strength and get a healthy extension stretch with extension exercises, which follow in the next section.

Back Extension That Helps Reduce Back Pain

Back extension exercises are a mainstay of back strengthening and pain-reduction programs. Back extension unloads lower back discs and is helpful to relieve the pain of damaged discs. More than an isolated exercise, it is important to practice the upper body movement needed to retrain away from a tight, forward-bent posture that is so damaging on the discs and muscles. Extension is different from the compressive loading of excess lordosis. You can feel the difference easily for yourself. Done properly, extension does not compress the spine or fold it under body weight.

- Lie face down, hands at your sides and off the floor. Lightly lift your upper body a few inches, then lower. Don't force. Don't crane your head back. Keep your head in line with your body. Start with one or two lifts. Gradually increase. Back extension done this way strengthens the back far better and in healthier ways than leaning over to lift weights.

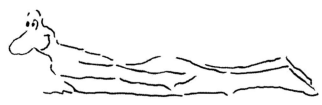

- To progress, move your arms out to the sides to add more weight to the lift. Then try with arms overhead. Don't force or yank. Lift with your muscles.

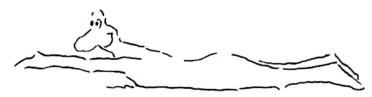

- For the lower back muscles, lie flat and lift one leg up from the floor, knees straight. Hold and lower several times. Switch legs and repeat. To progress, lift both legs together. Don't yank or force.

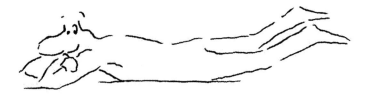

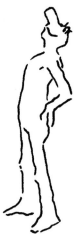

- In addition to extension exercise for strength, extension is an important stretch. It is different from letting the lower back compress backward all day under body weight in unhealthy overarching. During the day stretch your back and shoulders backward often, especially after sitting or working in poor bent forward positions (which you know not to do in the first place).

- Lean backward over your chair back. Make sure to get the upper back lifting backward, not just pinching your neck back. Better yet, get out of the chair.

At the minimum, do at least ten back extensions every day. Work up from there. If you aren't used to exercising your back muscles you may be sore at first. This is not injury; this is much-needed progress. If you feel muscles working, that is right. If you feel pinching or electric shock pain, don't continue the exercises. See your doctor. For some, tightness makes it uncomfortable to lie face down and extend back. Check the stretches for the chest on page 20 and for the hip on pages 44-46.

More extension exercises and others to relieve back and neck pain (and not get it in the first place) are in the second edition of the book "Health & Fitness in Plain English," by Dr. Jolie Bookspan. The book has thirty-one chapters on all aspects of fitness, nutrition, health, and joint pain. Another book with exercises and information for many different kinds of pain is "Fix Your Own Pain Without Drugs or Surgery." See the website: www.DrBookspan.com.

Arching Itself Isn't the Culprit

You are supposed to have a small inward curve in your lower back. In contrast, exaggerating the arch with upper body weight flopping downward, results in compressive loading. The two are often confused, giving rise to recommendations to some back pain patients to avoid all arching and sports requiring extension. Proper back extension, explained in the previous section, is important exercise for back health. Healthy extension lying down unloads the discs, and can be done without compressing the spine. Extending the upper body back during standing is needed in tennis, gymnastics, yoga, stretching, and other activities. Don't allow your lower back to arch and fold backward under your weight. By holding upper body weight up with abs, and getting back extension more from the upper spine, you can extend back without weight pressing down onto the lower back.

To see the difference between extending the spine and letting it pinch backward and compress in hyperlordosis try this:
- Stand up. Allow your back to arch, curving your abdomen out in front. Let upper body weight relax downward and backward until you feel the weight on your lower back. (Don't do this if you have back pain.) This is the arching that presses down on the lower back, making it ache. Tuck your hip under and pull the upper body straight to reduce the arch, as taught in pages 28-29 and used in all moves in this book. The pressure in the lower back should stop.

- Now begin to lean your upper body backward again. This time, lift upward and use abs to hold weight up and off your lower back. Keep holding upper body weight up as you extend the upper body backward, until you can look straight up, keeping neutral spine. Relax your shoulders and keep them back. It should be a good-feeling stretch with no pain.

- Lean backward again further, and add bending your knees to tilt further. Continue pulling forward with your abs, and don't allow your weight to slump backward. You should feel abdominal muscle exercise to prevent spine loading and no back pain.

Supported extension with roman chair exercise
Roman Chair lifts can be done either facing up for abdominal training or facedown for back muscle extension. There are various kinds of seats in gyms or you can make your own over a sturdy surface (or friend) to hold your legs and lower body. In up-facing Roman Chair, use supported extension:

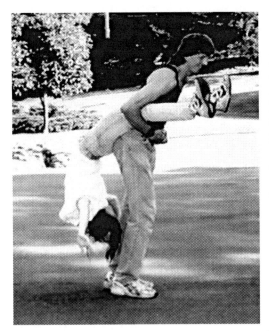

Strongly use your ab muscles to decelerate and counter your upper body weight pulling downward on your lower spine as you extend backward to support the extension.

To challenge ab muscles functionally, lift your upper body to horizontal position. Hold your body flat and straight without arching before repeating.

Supported arching with headstands and handstands
Use the ab-supported arch for headstands and handstands when you do them with the low back extended. Hold the weight of your legs up with your ab muscles, not your lower back joints.

Don't allow the weight of your legs to fold your lower back into an angle, compressing the facet joints and surrounding soft tissue.

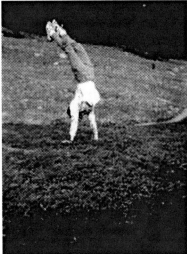

Practice using your abdominal muscles to hold healthy spine position for headstands and handstands. It is harder to balance and is more exercise to hold straight, which is one reason that people like to overarch. Practice straight position for better abdominal strength plus balance training.

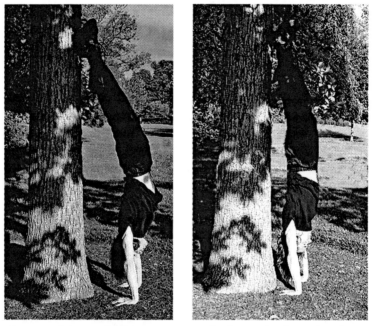

Left: Over-arching, which compresses the lower back under the weight of the legs. Right: Reducing the arch to straighten the body, reduce lower back compression, and increase abdominal workout.

Other activities
In many activities, you need to extend back but still not compress the lower spine. Use good abdominal muscle technique to keep upper body weight lifted up and off the lower back to prevent the your lower spine from being compressed. Prevent allowing upper body weight to just sink downward against the lower spine while leaning back for windsurfing, water skiing, for "hiking out" to counterbalance sailboats in the wind, to dodge flying objects and fists, to dip while ballroom dancing, to take photographs from certain angles, for doing the limbo dance, and to reach awkward overhead repairs.

Avoiding Back Pain When Sitting

Check to see if you tuck the hip too much when sitting. The rounding that results from too much hip tuck can make your back hurt, and can eventually push discs outward. Over time, the discs can degenerate, even herniate. Disc damage is not a disease; it is a mechanical process that is easy to prevent and reverse. Discs are living parts that can heal, if you let them.

When sitting, keep the normal small inward curve of the lower back. Chairs and seats are often overly rounded outward—not good for healthy sitting. Put a small spacer, often called a "lumbar roll," in the outward curving space of the seat back. A small towel, shirt, or pair of gloves can work as well or better than an expensive commercial lumbar roll. If the roll is uncomfortable, it is usually too big or not properly placed.

To see the approximate size and placement of a lumbar roll, put your own hand in the space of your lower back. Lean upward and backward against your upper back. Do not round or push your lower back against the roll. You should feel relief from the pressure on your lower back when sitting as soon as you try it, if you are using it appropriately.

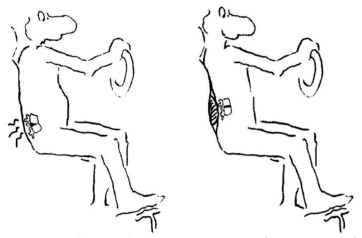

Left: injurious rounding. Right, maintaining neutral spine using a lumbar roll. Lean the upper body back against the seat, not the lower back against the roll.

What Are All the Muscles Called?

Ab muscles are named for their layout in your body—where they connect to bones and to each other. They don't work separately in real life. They work in combinations. That is why it is important to learn to use them together in functional exercises as described in this book.

Rectus abdominis

The muscle straight up the front of your abdomen is your rectus abdominis, which in Latin means "the straight abdominal." Your rectus abdominis starts on the front of your pelvic bone (lower front hipbone) and runs up to attach to where your middle ribs (fifth, sixth, and seventh) come together in front. Not all the rectus fibers run up the muscle. There are three, sometimes four intersections across it. You can see these lines in trim people. Contracting your rectus abdominal muscle pulls your ribs and hips toward each other to bend you forward or prevent arching backward. Holding your body upright while preventing backward arching is how the rectus abdominis (and other abdominal muscles) prevent the overarching that creates back pain. The rectus muscle does not automatically support your posture or prevent pain by any tightening or by virtue of being strong, in itself. Pain prevention is simple, by using the abdominal muscles to position your spine away from painful compressive slumping.

Obliquus externus

"Oblique" means slanted or not straight. Your oblique abdominal muscles run diagonally across your sides. If you put your fingertips at the top of your pants pockets, your hands line up in the direction of the outer set called external obliques. External oblique muscles begin as broad muscles on each side of your lower eight ribs. The outer external obliques on each side fuse together in a tough band in a nice line down the front of you your body, under your front or rectus muscle. The deeper external oblique fibers run almost straight down to your hipbones.

Your obliques work together in fun ways. When the external oblique fibers on your right side contract, they pull your right side closer to the middle of your pelvic bone so you twist to the left. You also use your right obliques to stay straight and resist forces that would twist or pull you to the right (for example, a dog leash or someone pulling you). When you contract your left external oblique, you twist to the right (or prevent turning your torso to the left). When you contract both, you bend forward or prevent bending backward. An important function they have when contracting together is to keep your hip from tilting forward in front. Preventing tilting and arcing is how your external oblique muscles help prevent back pain. Pain prevention comes from using your oblique muscles, not tightening or exercising them.

Obliquus internus

Your internal obliques lie under your external obliques in the opposite direction. If you cross your arms over your abdomen, your fingers assume the direction of the internal fibers. They begin at your hipbone and angle up and in to your lower three or four ribs.

Your right internal oblique contracts to pull the middle of your ribs to your right hip, twisting you to the right. The left internal oblique twists you to the left. The right external and left internal oblique work together to twist you left. The left external and right internal work together to twist right. Contracting them all helps you bend forward, prevent arching backward, and prevent your hip from tilting forward in front, which increases lordotic pressure on the lower spine. All the oblique muscles can resist forces that would make you want to slouch or twist in bad postures.

Transversus abdominis

Your innermost and thinnest abdominal muscle, the transversus, goes across your abdomen to help compress it for actions like breathing out fully, shouting, and childbirth. You can feel it when you breathe out as completely as you can. It is not the case that merely tightening the transversus like a girdle will prevent lower back injury when lifting or sitting. Although a popular assumption that the transversus must be tightened, Dr. Stuart McGill, one of the most important names in spine research, published that "drawing in" the abdominal muscles ("press the navel to spine") is detrimental to health of the lower back, and that tightening the abs impedes normal movement. In a paper in the *Archives of Physical Medicine Rehabilitation* (2007 Jan;88(1):54-62) he wrote, "There seems to be no mechanical rationale for using an abdominal hollow, or the transversus abdominis, to enhance stability."

More importantly, tightening will position your spine in the way that prevents injury. It will not prevent you from arching backward (or overly rounding forward) while lifting, either of which can injure your back. Back pain protection comes from repositioning your back by using, not tightening, all your abdominal muscles to prevent slouching into unfavorable angles. Moreover, when you hold the transversus tightly, you increase your blood pressure, and cannot breathe in fully or properly (belly breathing) because the major purpose of this muscle is to produce exhalation.

The transverse abdominus is usually one of the muscles that yogis tighten and involve in doing "locks" along with the pelvic floor muscles. It is sometimes asked in yoga and other classes if the TrA (transverse abdominus) is one of the pelvic floor muscles involved in genitourinary control, used to control urinary flow. The transverse abdominus is not part of the pelvic floor muscles to control continence. Ab strengthening is not needed for continence training. That does not mean that continence cannot be trained. It just uses other muscles. Train urinary continence by "holding" the stream. People sometimes tighten all the lower torso muscles when trying to figure out how to just control the urinary constrictor muscles. However, bladder control does not require any tightening of the abdominal muscles.

Using them all
You don't have to know the names of the muscles to use them. You don't have to tighten them. Just use them like other muscles to move your bones. Change your spine position away from arching back or sagging to the side during daily life and when you exercise. You will have better posture, prevent a major cause of lower back pain and injury, and get good core muscle exercise just by standing and moving properly.

Should You Work Your Abs Every Day or Every Other Day?

It is common to debate fiber type and fatigue to decide whether to exercise abdominal muscles daily or intermittently. Flurries of articles are written on which is correct.

What is missed is that, like your heart beating, you need your abdominal muscles working during all your movement. Doing crunches or any other ab exercise, then not using the abdominal muscles to control spine position the rest of the day; allowing upper body weight to press on your lower back, is missing the point of what abs are supposed to do. You are also missing an easy opportunity to burn calories, prevent back pain, and get a free all-day workout.

You may exercise your abs and still have back pain, no matter whether you exercised every day or every few days. Don't miss the point that abdominal muscles need to be in use all the time, not by tightening, but used just like any other skeletal muscles to move your bones into position. If you worked your abdominal muscles all the time to keep spine position healthy, you wouldn't need to go to a gym to do funny little crunches—not every day, nor every few days.

Why work out then allow overarching the rest of the day and undo all your efforts? Stand, sit, lift, and reach well all the time and you will exercise your abdominal and core muscles without stopping your day to go "work out."

Part III
Ab Devices, Potions, Gizmos

What About Ab Rocking Devices?

The various ab rocker devices on the market are little cages in various shapes to rock you for crunches. They attract users because they make crunches easy. The problems are all the same as with crunches.

Doing crunches with or without an ab device does not train you to use your abs in a way that you need for daily life. It is not a functional exercise. The crunching motion of the devices promotes the same round-shouldered, round-backed, hunched-over poor posture as crunches. This often occurs no matter how many instructions are given to keep the neck straight. It occurs even with devices that hold your neck up for you. Most people already stand, walk, and exercise round-shouldered. The last thing they need is to exaggerate and practice that bad posture as a deliberate exercise.

This entire book teaches ways to use your abs for good posture and effective use of abs during normal activity instead of crunches. Try the Ab Revolution exercises in this book instead. If you decide you must still do crunches, or if you are stuck in exercise classes that still do them, try this:

Save money on the device and use a dumbbell (or a book or other object). Instead of rounding your neck forward, put a dumbbell behind your low neck at the shoulder and press the back of your head onto the bar of the dumbbell as you lift up. The pressing activates muscles in the back of your neck. This activation quiets muscular activity in the front of your neck. It will help straighten your neck and stop the muscles in front of your neck from hurting.

It is still better not to crunches at all and to train your muscles in ways that strengthens more effectively, and trains the positioning that relives back pain, taught throughout this book.

What About Electronic Ab Zapper Belts?

"Watch TV while motorized stomach vibrator burns
more calories than 500 sit-ups a day"

"Use electronic stimulating muscle contractor to get
more muscle contractions than hundreds of sit ups"

Many advertisements for abdominal devices sound good, but are they true?

Early abdominal devices were little more than vibrators. They do not burn extra calories. Advertisers made claims comparing the relative number of calories you would burn in a longer time to a shorter one. In two hours of sitting in front of the television wearing the device, you would burn more calories than during the theoretical 15 to 30 minutes it would take to do the sit-ups, with or without a vibrator strapped to your abdomen. Burning calories is just your normal metabolism at work.

Other devices stem from electrical muscle stimulators (EMS) used in physical therapy to passively contract muscles atrophied from paralysis or wasting diseases. These devises have been around for a long time. There is muscle contraction but not enough to produce the results claimed.

What About Miracle Liquids and Fat Burners?

Many products on the market claim to make you burn fat while you sleep. Some products claim to give a workout so intense that you burn fat for hours after you finish exercising. Other products are pills tantalizingly called "fat burners."

First, everyone burns fat when they're asleep— and when they are awake too. Metabolizing stored fat is part of your round-the-clock energy production for body functions, whether you drink miracle potions or not. Advertising could just as honestly claim that if you stare at their special green dot you will burn calories in your sleep. But, don't pay money to buy the dot because you won't burn extra calories. You burn calories staring at a dot because you would burn calories anyway to breathe and live. You burn fat 24 hours a day as part of being alive.

When you exercise, no matter what device you use or what potion you drink, you increase your metabolism to meet energy needs. Metabolism slows to normal after you stop exercising, but takes a while to return to resting levels. Any product can truthfully claim to produce increased calorie burning after a workout. Just don't pay money for that because any nice run, bike, swim, or exercise will do the same.

Pills called "fat burners" are mostly stimulants. They do not selectively find your fat cells and eliminate them. Stimulants can have harmful effects from nervousness and grouchiness to heart trouble and inability to exercise safely in the heat. Regular use makes you unable to function well without them.

A good workout of dancing, skating, playing, biking, and other fun ways to move around will "pick you up" more effectively and safely than stimulants, will burn more calories, and keep you happier and healthier in the long run.

What About Neoprene Waist Bands?

Various products state that they "take off inches" just by wearing them. That have intriguing names like "waist support," "muscle support," "flab zapper," and "waist shrinker."

Commercial garments are simply a neoprene or other tight elastic band to wear around your waist (or thighs, or hips, or wherever). The band squeezes you, temporarily shrinking your circumference through simple compression.

The garments have nothing to do with toning or supporting the muscles, sweat loss, weight loss, or body fat loss. They just compress, temporarily. Have you ever noticed when you take off your socks, that there is a dent around your leg from the sock band? The elastic sock compressed your flesh leaving you temporarily smaller. Your leg returns to normal circumference quickly. The same thing happens with the neoprene waistbands. It is just a gimmick.

What About Ab Machines?

When using abdominal machines, check to make sure you don't use them in ways that don't use the abdominal muscles. If you allow your back to arch, your body weight hangs on your lower back vertebrae, causing back pain and reducing abdominal exercise.

To use ab machines so that you use your abdominal and core muscles, tuck your hips under as if beginning a crunch. Straighten your torso. You will immediately feel your abdominal muscles start to work. Pressure on the lower back will be relieved. For more effective, healthful, functional exercise, stay off your knees.

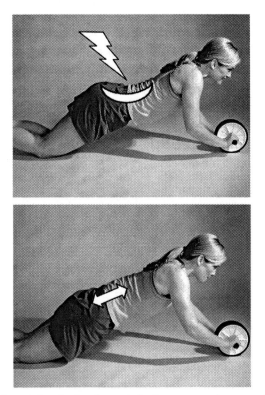

Top: Arched lower back. Body weight hangs on the vertebrae. Abs not in use. Bottom: Straightened posture. You will feel abs highly in use, and pressure relieved on the spine.

Instead of an expensive machine, you can use two roller skates, or a simple wheel, or a slippery floor with socks on your hands and feet.

One way to remind yourself of the hip tuck for using ab machines is to start on all fours and curl your back upward like a cat, feeling how your behind tucks and rotates downward (Method 5, page 28). Then see if you can tuck the hip without squeezing or tightening your gluteal muscles while using the ab machine. It is not tightening you want, but easily using ab muscles to move your spine out of unhealthful position to straight position. Keep your head up. Make sure your lower back does not sag or arch downward. Don't lift your behind upward; tuck it under. Use a mirror to watch your posture in side view.

The key point is to transfer the knowledge you just trained of how to change your spine position when doing the exercise, to when you are standing. Then you can stop painful overarching, using the hip tuck. You won't tuck so much that you round your back or stick your hips out in back. Use a mirror to watch your posture in side view.

What About Ab Isolators?

Several products on the market claim to better isolate your abdominal muscles and therefore somehow give you the abdomen pictured on the package. There is nothing in an isolating device that you cannot do without it. For instance, advertising for one device claims to hold your feet and legs in the specific position required for crunches. You can hold position yourself without the device, and it is still the same, bad, hunched-over posture that you don't want anyway.

Some of the devices add resistance to the abdominal exercises. More resistance increases the muscle activation you need to do the exercise, just like carrying extra packages adds more weight to your arms. There is nothing secret or scientific about doing more work to get more results. You can just hold a weight or your body weight, described in the Ab Revolution exercises in this book.

Dr. Steven Fleck, sport physiologist formerly with the U.S. Olympic Training Center, reminds us that "the value of these devices is their novelty. If they get you to exercise areas that you wouldn't normally exercise they might pay for themselves." Remember that the fine print on the packaging mentions that these products must be combined with healthy eating and regular exercise of all kinds. Moreover, they do not work your muscles the way you need or train you how to use them in daily activity.

Isolating a muscle is not helpful to your real life. Life is a multi-segment activity. Someone may have a muscular back from isolation exercises, yet injure themselves opening a window. Plenty of people run miles on treadmills, then sprain their ankle when walking on real earth. They are not used to using their body in a multi-functional, cooperative manner the way they need for real life. Similarly, people who do crunches in every workout and use every ab machine, often still stand with an arched spine, not using their abs.

How Do You Flatten Your Abdomen?

Use your abdominal muscles so that you do not curve your abdomen outward in unhealthful hyperlordotic spine. Check if you stand and exercise arched, so that you stand with your abdomen curved out. This is the opposite of having a flat abdomen.

No exercise selectively removes fat from a specific part, such as the abdomen, despite marketing claims. That myth is called "spot reducing." If spot reducing worked, people would have thin mouths from talking, speed skaters would have small legs, and the repeated act of chewing and swallowing large amounts of food would make your face thin.

Aerobic exercise burns fat. This fat comes from where it is stored. That means to lose fat, including fat from your abdomen, go out and have fun. Dance, run, swim, bike, row, skip, skate, jog, ski, run, walk, dig, play, and move in general. Weight training (including body weight training through Ab Revolution exercise) builds muscle, which burns more calories. Use the Ab Revolution exercises put together to make a full workout to burn more calories. Breathe, enjoy life, and instead of doing hated repetitions of exercises in unhealthful ways, get out and have fun using the positioning taught throughout this book.

Conventional abdominal exercise alone will not make you stand properly to prevent your lower back from arching with your abdomen sagging outward. It is not "sucking in" or tightening, but moving your torso into healthy position using the Ab Revolution for daily life.

How Do You Get a "Washboard?"

Bands of fibrous tissue called fascia run at intervals across your abdominal muscles. Doing abdominal exercise will enlarge the muscles enough to poke through the fascial bands giving a "washboard" or "ripple" or "six-pack" effect. However, the visual appearance of abdominal muscles does not mean a person is healthy, has strong muscles, or uses the ab muscles to hold healthful spine positioning to move in functional, healthy ways.

Use your muscles for real life outside of the gym—moving, balancing, lifting, reaching, and having fun. Consciously use your abs all the time to hold your spine without sagging into overarched hyperlordotic position.

Strong abdominal muscles that may not be apparent if body fat covers them. Don't diet in unhealthy ways just to get a cosmetic effect of abdominal muscles. Eat healthful meals. Cut out junk food. You will save money too. Keep moving in fun, healthful ways. Dieting without exercise may reduce visible fat, but leave you without the important healthful benefits of exercise and movement.

The next time you are standing and notice that your lower back hurts, check if you are standing hyperlordotic—overarching in a way that is hurting your back by not using your ab muscles. Notice if you are letting your body weight, and the weight of all you lift and carry, press down on your lower back. Check if your belt or waistband tilts downward in front and up in back instead of holding neutral spine. Use your abs to tilt your hip back under you and level your beltline, to lift your weight up and off your lower back and regain neutral spine.

Use The Ab Revolution to retrain your body to use your muscles without going to a gym. You will burn more calories. You will be straighter and taller. You will save your back. You will get more effective and functional exercise. You will exercise your brain. You will get a free, continuous, all-day workout.

It's a revolution.

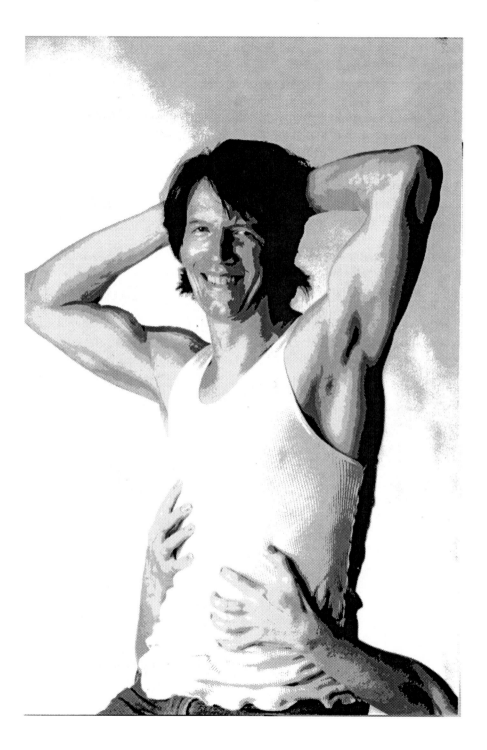

What Aerobics Instructors and Personal Trainers Say About Dr. Bookspan's Ab Revolution™

This class dispelled many myths about abs. I've learned many exercises to bring to my group fitness classes.
—*Jack Sannino, Group Exercise Instructor*

The Ab Revolution is a whole new way of life and a better way of doing abs. I have already reduced my own back pain. Great new method.
—*Mary Ann Rahman, Aerobics Teacher*

I liked this method. It is energetic, fun, and makes excellent functional sense. I've learned how to use my abs, for every day, all day.
—*Tracy Selekman, National Strength & Conditioning Association (NSCA) Certified Personal Trainer*

Excellent knowledge and workout on abs. The Ab Revolution already helped my back pain. I will have less trouble with my lower back during training now at age 62. Valuable information that I can pass on to our students.
—*Eb Molesch, 7th Degree Black Belt*

Books by Dr. Jolie Bookspan - see the website www.DrBookspan.com

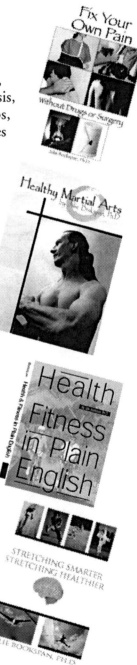

Fix Your Own Pain
Without Drugs or Surgery
Neck pain, back pain, shoulder, knee, foot, ankle, and hip pain, fasciitis, disc pain, sciatica, lordosis, flat feet, carpal tunnel, pinched nerve, cramps, hamstring, wrist—it's all here, with fun stories from real patients.

Healthy Martial Arts
Huge wealth of information for all athletes. Innovative training without injury. 232 pages. Over 200 photos. $24.95. Beautiful print edition and full color e-book. Winner of the Eastern USA International Black Belt Hall of Fame Reader's Choice Award.

Health & Fitness in Plain English
Second edition. Thirty-one fun chapters on exercise, fitness, nutrition, health, joint pain, and funny facts about your body and health. 371 pages, illustrated. $24.95 (US) ISBN: 1-58518-642-2

Stretching Smarter Stretching Healthier.
Fun, easy to read, immediately helpful techniques. $11.95. 106 pages. Over 200 humorous illustrations guide you step-by-step.

Diving Physiology in Plain English
The book for every scuba diver
246 pages, illustrated. New edition with
new blue cover. $40.00. Published by
the Undersea and Hyperbaric
Medical Society (UHMS)

**Diving and Hyperbaric Medicine
Review For Physicians**
Reviews the entire field, including
Sample board exam questions and
answers. 226 pages. $50.00

**Hyperbaric Medical Review For Certified
Hyperbaric Technologist
(CHT) and Certified Hyperbaric
Registered Nurse (CHRN)**
All chamber and nursing topics,
TCom module, sample certification
questions and answers. Prepares you for
the board exam.190 pages. $40.00

Credits

Cover model Paul Plevakas
Cover photo Julia Lehman, Vision13 Photography
Roman chair photo Wowk Photography
Author photo Robert Troia Photography
Illustrations by Todd Sargood and Jolie Bookspan Plevakas
Some images © 2006, Jupiterimages Corporation
2nd edition edits to prepare for 3rd edition, Thomas H. Kohn, Esq.
Photo models for exercises are Dr. Bookspan's dedicated hard-working students. If you see yourself and are not mentioned here, get in touch:

> Shelly Anthony
> Regina Basile
> Cynthia Brown
> Emily Canon
> Louis Costa
> Dr. Martin Dembitzer
> Angela and Andrea Fleegle
> Elsa Leung
> Rhonda McJeff
> Stacia Mellbourne
> Travis Mesman
> Jim Passio
> Sara Rathfon
> Danielle Tobin

About the Author

Dr. Jolie Bookspan knows abs. A career military scientist, she has a black belt in karate and was undefeated in the ring as a full contact Muay Thai kickboxer. After serving in the Army, she was research physiologist for the United States Navy, studying survival in extreme environments from undersea to climbing mountains to outer space—an interest that began as a child when she sat barefoot in the snow watching her grandfather and father go ice swimming every day. As a scientist, she has carried gear up and down the mountains and deserts of India, Nepal, Asia, and Northern Africa; swam to work in an underwater laboratory; was advisor to The Discovery Channel and police and military training departments, and was professor of anatomy at a college in the mountains of Mexico, where the entrance exam was getting up there without a nosebleed. Left paralyzed after breaking her back, neck, and most of everything else in an accident, she rehabbed using her own methods. She started over again as a white belt and earned her black belt a second time. Jolie and her husband Paul were inducted into the International Black Belt Hall of Fame and were the Eastern USA Martial Arts Association Man and Women of the Year 2004. Harvard clinicians have called Jolie "The St. Jude of the Joints" in her research and practice in sports medicine. Her pioneering methods are used around the world. She doesn't do crunches.

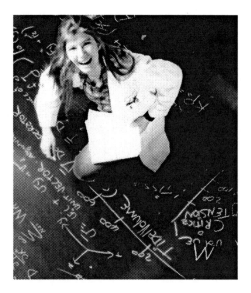

LaVergne, TN USA
15 September 2010
197116LV00010B/130/A